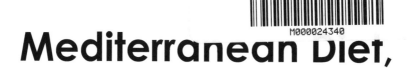

Mediterranean Diet,

Anti inflammatory Diet,

Alkaline Diet:

The ultimate guide for weight loss, find out how to lose weight with 3 diets

3 Books in 1

GILLIAN WILLET

Mediterranean Diet for Beginners

A diet plan, for meals prep, with 7 practical recipes throughout the week

To lose weight, live healthy and fit

GILLIAN WILLET

Table of Contents

Introduction

The Mediterranean diet is the name that has been given to a particular dietary regimen that was originally used by people in poorer regions of Italy and Greece for many centuries. This diet was not originally thought to be particularly healthy in these regions, as the people ate these foods because of necessity, rather than because of the Mediterranean diet weight loss and excellent nutrition benefits they experienced. This type of cuisine is far different from what you might expect from this region, but it is overall much healthier because things like lard and butter are rarely used.

In recent years, a growing number of men and women in different countries around the world have become increasingly concerned about their health. Because of the fact that many people have become more concerned about their overall health, these men and women have paid closer attention to what they eat on a regular basis. In the final analysis, these men and women are making dietary decisions designed to improve their general health and wellbeing.

As people have become more conscious of their health and diet, a considerable number of these same men and women have become interested in the Mediterranean diet regimen. If you are, in fact, a person who appreciates the interrelationship between diet and health, you may have a definite interest in the history of the Mediterranean diet regimen.

Before you can appropriately understand what the Mediterranean diet is all about, you need to appreciate that it is more of a concept than a specific dining routine. In reality, there is no such thing as a Mediterranean diet common to all of the countries in the Mediterranean region of the world. Rather, the "Mediterranean diet" consists of those food items that people who live in the various nations in the region consume in common.

Chapter One

History Of The Mediterranean Diet

The Mediterranean Diet is steeped in the culinary traditions of the Mediterranean region, particularly Greece and Italy. The importation of the diet into America and other parts of the world began in the 1940s and '50s.

The Mediterranean tradition offers a cousine rich in colors, aromas and memories, which support the taste and the spirit of those who live in harmony with nature. Everyone is talking about the Mediterranean diet, but few are those who do it properly, thus generating a lot of confusion in the reader.

And so for some it coincides with the pizza, others identified it with the noodles with meat sauce, in a mixture of pseudo historical traditions and folklore that do not help to solve the question that is at the basis of any diet: combine and balance the food so as to satisfy the qualitative and quantitative needs of an individual and in a sense, preserves his health through the use of substances that help the body to perform normal vital functions.

The purpose of our work is to demonstrate that the combination of taste and health is a goal that can be absolutely carried out by everybody, despite those who believe that only a generous caloric intake can guarantee the goodness of a dish and the satisfaction of the consumers. That should not be an absolute novelty, since the sound traditions of the Mediterranean cuisine we have used for some time in a wide variety of tasty gastronomic choices, from inviting colors and strong scents and absolutely in line with health.

The Mediterranean diet has its origins in a portion of land considered unique in its kind, the Mediterranean basin, which historians call "the cradle of society," because within its geographical borders the whole history of the ancient world took place.

The origins of the "Mediterranean Diet" are lost in time because they sink into the eating habits of the Middle Ages, in which the ancient Roman tradition - on the model of the Greek - identified in bread, wine and oil products a symbol of rural culture and agricultural (and symbols elected of the new faith), supplemented by sheep cheese, vegetables (leeks, mallow, lettuce, chicory, mushrooms), little meat and a strong preference for fish and seafood (of which ancient Rome was very gluttonous).

The rich classes loved the fresh fish (who ate it mostly fried in olive oil or grilled) and seafood, especially oysters, eaten raw or fried. Slaves of Rome, however, was destined to eat poor food consisting of bread and half a pound of olives and olive oil a month, with some salted fish, and rarely a little meat.

The Origins of the Mediterranean Diet

The concept of the Mediterranean diet is derived from the eating habits and patterns of the people who populate the countries of Italy, Greece, Spain, France, Tunisia, Lebanon and Morocco. As a result, the Mediterranean diet actually includes a tremendous array of delectable food. In point of fact, if a person elects to adopt the concept of the Mediterranean dining scheme, or if a person elects to follow a Mediterranean diet regimen, he or she will have the ability to enjoy a remarkable assortment of scrumptious fare.

The diet of the peoples that have populated the regions around the Mediterranean Sea actually have remained nearly completely unchanged for well over one thousand years. The history of the region is replete with examples of men and women living longer than similarly situated people who consumed alternate diets. Through the centuries, the people of the Mediterranean Sea region have enjoyed longer lives that people in other parts of the world at the same historical epoch.

At the heart of the Mediterranean diet are foods and beverages that are indigenous to the geographic landmass surrounding the Mediterranean Sea. In short, the development of the Mediterranean dieting and dining pattern initially developed by providence. The people of the region naturally and understandably ate those foods and drank those beverages that readily were available in and around their homes.

The Historical Elements of the Mediterranean Diet Scheme

As mentioned previously, over the centuries, the diet of the peoples of the Mediterranean Sea region has remained essentially unchanged. The Mediterranean diet consists of the bountiful consumption of a number of healthy food items including:

* Fresh fruit

* Fresh vegetables

* Low fat nuts

* Whole grains

* Monounsaturated fat

In a similar vein, the Mediterranean diet utilized by people for generation after generation excludes or limits certain food items that have been deemed harmful in recent scientific studies. These less than desirable food items include:

* Saturated fats

* Red and fatty meat

* Rich dairy products

* Fatty fish

Chapter Two

The Mediterranean Diet

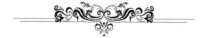

By its name alone, the Mediterranean diet attracts a lot of current and would be dieters due to its exotic name. But what is it exactly? One concern of the Mediterranean diet is that it allows 40% fat consumption. Let's go into more detail as it seems a waste to just let it go without giving it a fair reading.

The Mediterranean diet evolved from the respective diets of countries surrounding the Mediterranean basin. Among the countries surrounding the basin are the south of France, southern Italy, Spain, Portugal, Greece and Cyprus. Based on scientific data, people around the Mediterranean basin had lower rates of cardiovascular disease compared to Americans who, for all intents and purposes, consumed the same relative amount of fat.

One possible explanation is the presence of olive oil and red wine. Olive oil lowers cholesterol levels in the blood, while red wine contains flavonoids. Flavonoids are anti-oxidants that also help the body when dealing with allergenic material, viruses and cancer causing agents.

Another contributing factor to a European's better health could be the fact that they tend to walk more than Americans do. Questions have also been raised as to whether the Mediterranean diet contributes enough iron and calcium to the diet. Green vegetables and goat cheese have been found to contribute these nutrients respectively.

The thing about the Mediterranean diet is that its foods are often rich and tasty thanks to olive oil. Normally, margarine and hydrogenated oils lack the flavor that olive oil gives out. Another part of the diet is regular but moderate consumption of red wine. Saturated fat consumption is low as opposed to high amounts of monounsaturated fat and dietary fiber. This is due to the fact that the diet includes big servings of fruits, vegetables, breads, cereals, olive oil and fish.

Characteristically speaking, the Mediterranean diet has high consumption of olive oil. Breads, cereals, fruits and vegetables likewise have a high rate of consumption in the diet. Fish and poultry as well as wine are moderately consumed, while eggs and red meat are rated as very low in consumption.

The problem with most diets is that they tend to be extreme. Some diets, like the vegetarian diet, limit a person to just eating fruits, tofu, yogurt and vegetables. Other diets would require high protein intake while severely limiting intake of the other food groups. Like a user friendly computer, the Mediterranean diet does not go to extremes to achieve a desired result. The diet allows for consumption of tasty foods. This allows the dieter to actually enjoy the gastronomic delights normally prohibited by other diets. A solid testament to this fact rests on the presence of wine in the diet.

The most surprising aspect of the Mediterranean diet is that fat is regarded as a healthy dietary component. Keep in mind that it is the fat that gives food most of its flavor. Two substances, omega-3 fatty acids and monounsaturated fats, are considered to be healthy and are not restricted in the diet. Olive oil, canola oil and nuts are good sources of monounsaturated fat while fish, vegetables and nuts contain the healthy omega-3 acids.

Saturated fats and trans-fat, on the other hand are considered to be unhealthy as they contribute to heart disease. Red meat, butter cheese and milk are sources of saturated fat while processed foods contain hydrogenated oils from which trans-fat comes from.

The Mediterranean diet emphasizes: Eating primarily plant-based foods, such as fruits and vegetables, whole grains, legumes and nuts. Replacing butter with healthy fats such as olive oil and canola oil and using herbs and spices instead of salt to flavor foods.

FAST FACTS ABOUT THE MEDITERRANEAN DIET

There is no one Mediterranean diet. It consists of foods from a number of countries and regions including Spain, Greece, and Italy.

The Mediterranean diet is a great way to replace the saturated fats in the average American diet.

There is an emphasis on fruits, vegetables, lean meats, and natural sources.

It is linked to good heart health, protection against diseases such as stroke, and prevention of diabetes.

Moderation is still advised, as the diet has a high fat content.

The Mediterranean diet should be paired with an active lifestyle for the best results.

The Mediterranean diet is a way to ensure food comes from a range of natural, healthful sources.

The Mediterranean diet consists of:

- High quantities of vegetables, such as tomatoes, kale, broccoli, spinach, carrots, cucumbers, and onions

- Fresh fruit such as apples, bananas, figs, dates, grapes, and melons.
- High consumption of legumes, beans, nuts, and seeds, such as almonds, walnuts, sunflower seeds, and cashews
- Whole grains such as whole wheat, oats, barley, buckwheat, corn, and brown rice
- Olive oil as the main source of dietary fat, alongside olives, avocados, and avocado oil
- Cheese and yogurt as the main dairy foods, including Greek yogurt
- Moderate amounts of fish and poultry, such as chicken, duck, turkey, salmon, sardines, and oysters
- Eggs, including chicken, quail, and duck eggs
- Limited amounts red meats and sweets
- Around one glass per day of wine, with water as the main beverage of choice and no carbonated and sweetened drinks

This focus on plant foods and natural sources means that the Mediterranean diet contains nutrients such as:

Healthful fats: The Mediterranean diet is known to be low in saturated fat and high in monounsaturated fat. Dietary guidelines for the United States recommend that saturated fat should make up no more than 10 percent of calorie intake.

Fiber:

The diet is high in fiber, which promotes healthy digestion and is believed to reduce the risk of bowel cancer and cardiovascular disease.

High vitamin and mineral content:

Fruits and vegetables provide vital vitamins and minerals, which regulate bodily processes. In addition, the presence of lean meats provides vitamins such as B-12 that are not found in plant foods.

Low sugar:

The diet is high in natural rather than added sugar, for example, in fresh fruits. Added sugar increases calories without nutritional benefit, is linked to diabetes and high blood pressure, and occurs in many of the processed foods absent from the Mediterranean diet.

It is difficult to give exact nutritional information on the Mediterranean diet, since there is no single Mediterranean diet. This is because a variety of cultures and regions is involved.

Benefits

The Mediterranean diet is not specifically a weight loss diet, but cutting out red meats, animal fats, and processed food may lead to weight loss.

In areas where the diet is consumed, there are lower rates of mortality and heart disease, and other benefits.

Diabetes

The Mediterranean diet can help protect people from type 2 diabetes and improve glycemic control.

Several studies have shown that those who follow a Mediterranean diet have lower fasting glucose levels that those do not.

Basically, a Mediterranean diet calls for people to eat a great deal of fresh fruit, plant foods, fish, poultry, some dairy products, while using extra virgin olive oil as the primary source of fat. Also, a moderate amount of eggs can be eaten each month, while red meat is to be avoided as much as possible. Red meat can be eaten in low amounts, but meals should not be centered around it because of how it affects the heart.

The Mediterranean diet is meant to lower the risk of heart disease, since olive oil is high in monounsaturated fats, which have been known to reduce this risk substantially. This also reduces the body's cholesterol levels, which is also a positive thing for the body.

THE CONCEPT OF THE MEDITARRANEAN FOOD PYRAMID

For most of us, the most recognized symbol of healthy food is found in the food pyramid. It indicates which foods we should eat in which portion sizes so that our body receives the nutrients it requires. If you're creating a healthy diet plan you would do well to look at the Mediterranean diet food pyramid. The Mediterranean diet is recognized as one of the healthiest diets in the world and is actually endorsed by the Mayo Clinic.

What is the Mediterranean Diet Food Pyramid?

The Mediterranean diet food pyramid is an alternative to the traditional one which is becoming increasingly popular because it is not based on popular food trends. The diet itself is founded on thousands of years of tradition within the Mediterranean region. The dietary traditions of Mediterranean countries have long been recognized as very healthy, and the food that they consume is one of the main factors in that healthiness. Knowing the difference between the traditional food pyramid and the Mediterranean one will assist you in improving your health.

The Mediterranean diet food pyramid is significantly different to the traditional one with which we are familiar. There are certain glaring differences, namely;

- The Mediterranean one does not have a fats category
- Red meat is at the top of the Mediterranean pyramid as a food to eat least of all along with sweets/desserts.

- Olive oil is grouped with the fruits and vegetables as something to be consumed frequently

The top portion of the Mediterranean diet food pyramid starts with red meat as a source of animal protein. Red meat and sweets are the least consumed foods in the Mediterranean, around 2-3 times per month. The next category, consumed a couple of times per week, are poultry, eggs and dairy products like cheese and yogurt. Next comes fish and seafood which are consumed almost daily. Basically, the Mediterranean diet is low in saturated fats and high in monounsaturated fats and omega 3.

The bottom level of the pyramid is composed of fruits, vegetables, legumes (beans), nuts, seeds, herbs, spices, whole grain bread, whole grain pasta, couscous, brown rice, polenta and other whole grains. People in the Mediterranean rarely eat processed grains (i.e. white flour). A large variety of these fresh foods are eaten daily, and they are usually either raw or lightly cooked. This means that the nutrients are still intact. Cooking foods actually kills most nutrients or renders them undigestible. Hence, it is always better to eat food raw or partially cooked.

The final part of the Mediterranean pyramid is the recommendation of six glasses of water per day and a moderate amount of wine (i.e. one glass of red wine with dinner).

It is interesting to note that olive oil is grouped with the fruit and vegetables in the Mediterranean pyramid. As you can imagine, olive oil is a large part of the Mediterranean diet and many dishes contain it. While it is true that oil is high in calories, olive oil is a healthy monounsaturated fat which is high in antioxidants and contains omega 3 so we can consume a little more as long as we don't go overboard.

Monounsaturated oils like olive oil are anti-inflammatory and are good for diseases like asthma and arthritis. They're also heart healthy because the omega 3 lowers LDL ("bad") cholesterol, and raises HDL ("good") cholesterol. The most healthy olive oil is extra virgin olive oil.

You may be wondering how people in the Mediterranean receive their iron since they don't eat a lot of red meat. The answer to this is the same as it would be for a vegetarian. Legumes (beans) and green leafy vegetables are also good sources of iron and the Mediterranean diet is full of these healthy foods. In fact, the whole Mediterranean diet food pyramid consists of healthy foods ensuring that those who follow the Mediterranean diet experience optimum health.

Mediterranean Food Pyramid

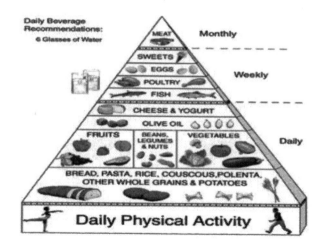

The main concepts of the Food Pyramid are the "proportionality", that is the right amount of foods to choose from for each group, the "portion" standard quantity of food in grams, which is assumed as the unit of measurement to be a balanced feeding, the "variety", i.e., the importance of changing the choices within a food group, and "moderation" in the consumption of certain foods, such as fat or sweets.

As you can see, at the base of the pyramid are grains, followed by fruits and vegetables, legumes, olive oil, low-fat cheese and yogurt, which should be eaten daily. Meat is not excluded, but is given the preference to that of chicken, rabbit and turkey rather than beef. Along with fish and eggs should be eaten only a few times a week, for the supply of high quality protein. Beef or red meat should be eaten only a few times a month.

Each group includes foods, which are substantially "equivalent" on the nutritional plan, in the sense that they provide nearly the same type of nutrients. It is obvious that, within the same group, foods despite being homogeneous with each other can have small differences in terms of quality and quantity of patrimony in nutrients.

However, this does not affect the concept of "interchangeability" of foods. The latter in fact, if they belong to the same group, being nutritionally equivalent, may be substitutes for each other, without, however, affecting the adequacy of the diet, provided you comply with the variety. In nature does not exist a "complete" food, i.e. it contains all the nutrients the body needs, and that is why it is necessary to vary as much as possible food choices and properly combine foods from the different groups.

A very varied diet not only avoids the risk of nutritional imbalances and possible consequent metabolic imbalances, but it also satisfies the taste of fighting the monotony of flavors. Each group expected is represented by at least a portion of the foods that constitute it, to vary the choices within the same group.

Understanding The Mediterranean Diet

The Mediterranean Diet is not a diet per se but a loose term referring to the dietary practices of the people in the Mediterranean region. Each country that borders the

Mediterranean Sea offers a variant to the Mediterranean Diet. Differences in ethnic background, culture, agricultural production, and religion between the Mediterranean countries creates the variation in each country's diet. However, each diet offers a number of characteristics that are common to all of the Mediterranean countries.

The Mediterranean Diet has a high consumption of fruits, vegetables, beans, nuts, seeds, bread, and other cereals. Traditionally, fruits and vegetables are locally grown in the Mediterranean Diet. Fruits and vegetables often are consumed raw or minimally processed. Fruits and vegetables contain many essential vitamins and minerals as well as antioxidants that are crucial for good health.

The Mediterranean Diet's primary source of fat is in the form of a monounsaturated fat. Olive oil is a monounsaturated fat that is a rich source of antioxidants including vitamin E. Olive oil is used instead of butter, margarine, and other fats. In fact, butter and cream are only used on special occasions. Olive oil in the

Mediterranean Diet is used to prepare tomato sauces, vegetable dishes, salads, and to fry fish.

The Mediterranean Diet encourages moderate intake of fish but little to no intake of meat. Red meat and poultry are consumed only sparingly. Fish is the meat of choice. About 5-15 oz. of oily fish, in particular are consumed weekly. Oily fish includes tuna, mackerel, salmon, trout, herring, and sardines. Oily fish are a great source of omega-3 fatty acids.

Dairy products are consumed in low to moderate amounts. Dairy products from a variety of animals such as goats, sheep, buffalo, cows, and camels are primarily consumed in the form of low fat cheese and yogurt. Very little fresh milk is consumed. Meals are usually accompanied by wine or water.

The Mediterranean Diet encourages low to moderate consumption of wine. Wine is usually consumed with a meal. The type of wine consumed is usually red wine which contains a rich source of phytonutrients. Among the phytonutrients, polyphenols especially are powerful antioxidants. Studies have shown that men and women who have a light to moderate consumption of alcohol live longer than nondrinkers. One alcoholic drink (1.5 oz. distilled spirits, 5 oz. wine, 12 oz. beer) daily for women and two alcoholic drinks daily for men is considered moderate intake of alcohol.

If you are looking to incorporate the Mediterranean Diet into your life, here are a few suggestions. Fruits and vegetables should be of a wide variety. You should try for at least 7-10 servings of whole fruits and vegetables daily. You should avoid any vegetables that are prepared in butter or cream sauces. High fiber breads, cereals, and pasta are consumed daily. This includes brown rice, bran, whole grain bread and cereal. You should avoid sweets, white bread, biscuits, breadsticks, and any refined carbohydrates.

Protein intake is low in saturated fat. Protein intake from red meat is of lean cuts, poultry without the skin, and low fat dairy foods (skim milk, yogurt). You should avoid bacon, sausage, and other processed or high fat meat. You should also avoid milk or cheese that is not low fat.

Intake of fish is 1-2 times weekly from oily fish, flaxseed, walnuts, and spinach. Healthy oils (extra virgin olive oil, canola oil, flaxseed oil) are used for cooking, salad dressings, and other uses. You should avoid omega-6 oils such as corn, sunflower, safflower, soybean, and peanut. Your diet should also include peas, beans, soybeans, lentils, tree nuts (almonds, pecans, walnuts, Brazil nuts), and legumes. You should avoid heavily salted or honey roasted nuts.

A moderate intake of alcohol with the evening meal is optional. The Mediterranean Diet emphasizes whole natural foods. This means avoiding fast food, fried food, margarine, chips, crackers, baked goods, doughnuts, or any processed foods that contain trans fatty acids.

The Mediterranean style diets are very close to the dietary guidelines of the American Heart Association. Diets of the Mediterranean people contain a relatively high percentage of fat calories, about 40%. The American Heart Association endorses a diet that contains about 30% fat intake. However, the average Mediterranean

Diet has less saturated fat than the average American diet.

Researchers are now trying to deduce the components of the Mediterranean Diet that are responsible for the Mediterranean populations' longer life expectancy compared to other European populations. However, the combined effects of different ingredients such as a relaxed eating attitude, plenty of sunshine, and more physical activity are likely to be contributing to the overall healthy lifestyle of the Mediterranean region. The Mediterranean Diet has a lower incidence of heart disease and cancer, which makes the Mediterranean Diet an overall good choice in health.

FOCUS OF THE MEDITERRANEAN DIET

The main focus of the Mediterranean Diet is actually on vegetables, fruit, unrefined carbohydrates such as root vegetables and wholegrain cereals (refined carbohydrates being things like bread, cakes, pasta and refined cereals). It is also high in fibre, and low in sugar and saturated fat. This describes the Mediterranean Diet in a nutshell. Once you successfully incorporate this in your routine, you certainly won't go wrong. Part of it is their approach to meat. The focus is less on red meat and more on poultry and seafood.

In general, people in the Mediterranean only eat red meat a few times per month but they eat poultry at least once per week and fish and seafood even more often. As you can imagine, this reduces their cholesterol levels significantly because of the Omega 3 in the fish, hence the reduction in heart disease risk. They also eat dairy products daily like goat's cheese and yogurt.

Quite obviously, lower cholesterol levels are the first step toward heart health. But where do we get cholesterol from? Cholesterol comes from saturated (bad) fats found in dairy foods and meats. Another contributing factor to heart disease is sodium (salt), although our body needs sodium, in western society we tend to consume too much sodium. As much as possible, avoid foods high in the saturated fats found in meat and dairy, when eating red meat, try to have lower fat options.

What is the Mediterranean diet's answer to this? The secret is food high in healthy polyunsaturated and monounsaturated fats like those found in seafood, and olive oil. These also contain plenty of Omega 3 fatty acids which actively reduce cholesterol levels. Omega 3 fatty acids are found in fatty fish. Popular varieties in the Mediterranean diet include sardines, whitebait, salmon, tuna, herring and mackerel. Other popular Mediterranean seafood choices include mussels, crab, shrimp, red mullet, squid, swordfish and sea bass.

There are many health benefits to following a Mediterranean diet. The people of the Mediterranean have a much lower incidence of cancer, heart disease, stroke, diabetes and even things like Alzheimer's as a result of their diet compared to those of us in western societies. All of these things lead to to living a long and healthy life.

The final secret of the Mediterranean diet is a healthy exercise regime. While most acknowledge the importance of exercise, very few people actually maintain a regular exercise routine. It doesn't have to be anything strenuous, a 20-30 minute walk per day is sufficient. But many of us are too lazy to do this, we'd rather rely on the car. Or we feel that we are too busy to find time to exercise. But think of it this way, if we don't find time, we'll LIVE less time!

Chapter Three

Why The Mediterranean Diet Is A Healthy Choice In The 21st Century-Nutritionist And Doctors Review

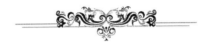

If you are a person who has been on the hunt for a solid diet plan, you may feel overwhelmed much of the time. In the 21st century it is nearly impossible for a person to turn on a television set or open a newspaper without being bombarded with advertisements for a variety of different diet plans and products.

With the tremendous array of diet plans, programs, supplements and aids on the market, it can seem nearly impossible to select a diet plan that can and will best meet your needs now and into the future. More importantly, it can be hard to discern if one or another of these various diet schemes actually is a healthy course to pursue. In many instances, fad diets really are not based on the fundamentals of healthy living.

As you go forward considering what type of diet plan or regimen will best serve your interests and improve your health into the future, you will want to take a look at the benefits that can be had through the Mediterranean diet.

While there are multiple reasons why the Mediterranean diet is a healthy approach, there are five primary reasons why the Mediterranean diet is a good choice.

1. The Benefits of Fruits, Vegetable, Fiber and Whole Grains

A major component of the Mediterranean diet includes the regular consumption of fresh fruits and vegetables. Medical experts and nutritionists universally agree that a person should eat between five and six servings of fresh fruits and vegetables (or steamed items) on a daily basis.

People who adhere to the Mediterranean diet actually end up eating more than the minimum recommended allowance of fruits and vegetables. As a result, nutritionists in different parts of the world have taken to recommending a Mediterranean based diet regimen to their clients. Similarly, doctors who consult with their patients about healthy eating practices oftentimes find themselves recommending the Mediterranean diet in this day and age.

Beyond fruits and vegetables, the Mediterranean diet includes healthy amounts of dietary fiber and whole grains. Fiber and whole grains have proven effective in lowering the incidence of heart disease and some types of cancer.

2. The Benefits of Olive Oil -- Avoiding Saturated Fat

Some people have a fundamental misperception about the Mediterranean diet. These people have heard that the Mediterranean diet is high in fat. On some level, there is some truth in the conception that the Mediterranean diet is higher in fat than are some other dieting programs. A person following the Mediterranean diet does take in about thirty percent of his or her daily calories from fat. (Most diets recommended the intake of calories from fat at the rate of about thirteen to fifteen percent per day. However, these diets are contemplating the ingesting of animal fat.)

The vast majority of fat that a person on the Mediterranean diet consumes comes from olive oil. In other words, the fat found in the Mediterranean diet is not the dangerous saturated fat that can cause disease, obesity and other health concerns. In fact, research has demonstrated that there are a number of solid benefits to consuming olive oil, including a reduction of the risk of the incidence of breast cancer in women.

3. Dairy in Moderation

While the consumption of low or non-fat dairy products in moderation can be beneficial in some instances, many people the world over rely on heavy creams, eggs and other fat filled dairy products in their daily diets. The Mediterranean diet is low in dairy. Indeed, any dairy products that actually are included within the diet regimen is low fat. A person is considered an extremely heavy egg eater if he or she consumes four eggs in a week.

4. Red Meat in Moderation

Very little red meat is included within the Mediterranean diet. When it comes to meat items, this diet relies on moderate amounts of lean poultry and fresh fish. As a result, people who follow the Mediterranean diet plan have lower levels of "bad" cholesterol and higher levels of "good" cholesterol.

In addition, because of the inclusion of lean, fresh fish in the diet, adherents to the Mediterranean diet enjoy the anti-oxidant benefits that are found in certain fish oils and products.

5. A Well Balanced Dieting Scheme

In the final analysis, the Mediterranean diet is gaining acclaim from experts and adherents the world over because it is a balanced dieting program. Study after study demonstrate that a balanced diet that is low in fat and that includes fruits, vegetable, whole grains and lean meat works to ensure total health and wellness.

In recent years, doctors, researchers, scientists and nutritionists have taken a close look at the Mediterranean diet. Nearly universally, these experts and professionals have come away from their examination of the Mediterranean diet with positive perceptions of the dieting scheme.

There are a number of reasons why experts of all sorts -- from doctors to researchers to nutritionists -- look favorable upon the Mediterranean diet regimen. By considering the benefits of the Mediterranean diet that have been identified by experts, you will be able to better determine if the Mediterranean diet is right for you.

1. Low in Saturated Fat

On the surface, a person giving only a cursory review of the Mediterranean diet might conclude that it is not a healthy diet plan because it is "high in fat." Concluding that the Mediterranean diet is high if fat and harmful is an erroneous conclusion.

While it is true that the Mediterranean diet does derive a significant percentage of its calories from fat (around thirty percent daily in most instances), the calories come primarily from olive oil and consist of unsaturated fats. In other words, being low in saturated fat, doctors are recommending the Mediterranean diet for their patients.

2. A Plentiful Array of Fresh Fruits and Vegetables

Doctors are recommending that their patients eat at least six servings of fruits and vegetables throughout the course of the day. Many of these same doctors are turning to the Mediterranean diet because as a matter of routine people who follow this diet program are eating more than the minimum recommended daily allowance of fruits and vegetables. Additionally, rather than using processed fruits and vegetables, the Mediterranean diet features an abundance of fresh fruits and vegetables.

3. Low in Red Meat

Many doctors can be found encouraging their patients to limit the amount of red meat that they include in their diets. Limiting red meat in a diet can assist in lowering the levels of "bad cholesterol," helping to reduce the indigence of heart disease and some cancers.

4. Low in Fatty Dairy Products

Another reason that doctors favor the Mediterranean diet is found in the fact that the diet plan is low in the consumption of fatty dairy products. More and more doctors are encouraging their patients to use only low fat or non fat dairy products. People who follow the Mediterranean diet actually use very little dairy on a day to day basis. For example, a heavy egg eater on the Mediterranean diet eats four eggs a week. Many do not eat eggs at all.

In addition, milk is used within the diet in limited fashion. Heavy creams and sauces are not on the Mediterranean menu at all.

5. Helpful in Preventing Diseases

One of the primary reasons that doctors recommend the Mediterranean diet for their patients rests in the fact that the diet program has been demonstrated as being helpful in reducing the risks of certain diseases, including:

- Cancer

- Heart disease
- Cardiovascular disease
- Hypertension
- Diabetes
- Obesity

6. A Ready Source of Fiber and Whole Grain

Finally, doctors recommend the Mediterranean diet for their patients because it is high in dietary fiber and whole grains. Both fiber and whole grains have proven important in preventing disease and in maintaining an overall sense of wellness and good health.

The main ingredient in a Mediterranean diet that is believed to have the most influence on a person's health is extra virgin olive oil. This is because the diet is inherently low in saturated fat, but the olive oil makes it high in monounsaturated fat, which (as previously mentioned) is good for your heart. The Mediterranean diet is also very high in dietary fiber, which promotes regularity of the digestive system. The diet can sometimes be high in salt, when is contains:

- Olives
- Capers
- Salad dressing
- Fish roe

This salt content is not necessarily a negative thing, however, because those items contain natural salts the body can use and absorb more comfortably.

Exercise

One thing that many people might not realize about Mediterranean diet weight loss is that the people who originated the diet generally worked outdoors and reaonably hard. This means they were getting plenty of exercise each and every day, in addition to fresh air. This, in combination with the small portions these individuals would eat, led to very lean and muscular bodies. This assisted heart health of course, which is another reason why they suffered far fewer deaths from cardiovascular problems.

Medical Findings

A number of medical studies have been conducted on the Mediterranean diet and they have found that men who lived in Crete, which is one of the regions where this diet was originally used, had a low incidence of heart disease. This occurred despite the fact they actually consumed high amounts of fats in many cases. One of the main reasons for this finding is that many of these men switched from butter to extra virgin olive oil because it was less expensive. They also had a high vitamin C intake and reduced the amount of red meat compared to other parts of the globe.

It should be noted that the findings of this study were so dramatic that the results were published before the study had been completed. This was because the people who were conducting the study did not believe they could keep the information to themselves any longer. Other diseases and illnesses which have been positively affected from this diet include osteoporosis, minimising the risk of some forms of cancer, allergies, alzheimers disease and there are more studies being undertaken.

Weight Loss

Further studies have shown instances of Mediterranean diet weight loss, as 322 people participated in an experiment where some people were subject to a low-carb diet, others undertook a low-fat diet, and some ate only a Mediterranean diet. The results showed that those who were on the Mediterranean diet had the greatest weight loss of all, with the top two participants losing 12 and 10 pounds respectively. The study highlighted that Mediterranean diet weight loss is effective and should be considered by anyone who is having trouble losing weight.

Chapter Four

Mediterranean Diet Health Benefits

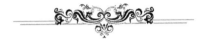

The Mediterranean diet has many health benefits. Wondering researchers have spent years trying to discover why. Although many regions have adopted a much more westernized diet habit which has resulted in a mounting obesity issue, communities that still follow the traditional Mediterranean diet continue to experience health which is the envy of the western world.

The Mediterranean diet consists primarily of fresh, healthy plant food like whole grains, vegetables, fruits, nuts, legumes, olives, fish and seafood. They combine this with reduced amounts of red meat and dairy products.

The Mediterranean diet is more nutritious because foods are less processed. Processing food, and even cooking it, deprives it of nutrients. But in a traditional Mediterranean diet, most foods are eaten raw or lightly cooked. When red meat is served it is usually trimmed of excess fat. The overall diet provides plentiful fiber, healthy fats, vitamins, minerals, protein and essential fatty acids required by the body to maintain health and prevent chronic illnesses like heart disease and cancer.

Another notable aspect of the traditional Mediterranean diet is that not every meal contains animal flesh (i.e. meat or fish). There are commonly days with no animal flesh being consumed at all. On these days, the protein portion of the meal is derived from things like beans, nuts, seeds and eggs. Although eggs are still animal products, recent research indicates that eggs do NOT increase blood cholesterol as scientists and doctors used to believe. Another modern day alternative to meat is tofu which comes from soy beans. While this is not a part of the diet, it would certainly be a worthwhile addition to it.

All of these things result in the Mediterranean diet being high in monounsaturated fatty acids, otherwise known as M.U.F.As which are healthy fats. Diets containing M.U.F.As (and polyunsaturated fats, or P.U.F.As) rather than saturated and trans fats, tend to provide certain health benefits including reduced risk of:

- Heart disease
- High Cholesterol
- Stroke
- Cancer
- Type II Diabetes
- Parkinson's Disease
- Alzheimer's
- Depression
- Metabolic syndrome

Lets take a closer look at these.

Reduced risk of heart disease and high Cholesterol

High levels of saturated fats result in increased cholesterol in the bloodstream. Over time, the cholesterol attaches to the walls of arteries causing a narrowing of the arteries that can lead to blockages, heart attacks and heart disease. Quite clearly, the reduced amount of saturated fat in traditional Mediterranean diets results in lower cholesterol levels. In some cases, high cholesterol is hereditary and is caused by the liver producing too much. A healthy diet containing high amounts of Omega 3 fatty acids is proven to actively combat this issue and can have a significant lowering effect on cholesterol levels.

Reduced risk of Diabetes

Consumption of complex carbohydrates and high fiber foods reduces the Glycemic Index of foods and low GI foods prevent spikes in blood sugar levels. So a low GI diet such as the Mediterranean diet tends to prevent diabetes. See the section on Metabolic syndrome below.

Reduced risk of Parkinson's & Alzheimer's

Some studies indicate that people who adhere to the Mediterranean diet have lower rates of Parkinson's and Alzheimer's diseases. Researchers are unsure why this is the case, but they believe that healthy food choices improving cholesterol, blood sugar levels and blood vessel health may be the cause.

Reduced risk of Depression

British Researchers studied depression and diet in more than 3,000 middle-aged office workers for five years. Their findings indicated that people who ate a diet high in processed meat, chocolate, sugar, fried food, refined cereals and high-fat dairy products were more likely to suffer depression. But people who ate a diet rich in fruits, vegetables and fish similar to a Mediterranean diet were less likely to suffer depression. Their findings support other research that has found that healthy diets can protect against disease.

Reduced risk of Metabolic syndrome

Many overweight and obese people suffer from a condition called Metabolic Syndrome. Metabolic syndrome is a group of conditions - high blood pressure, a abnormal blood sugar levels, excessive body fat around the waist or abnormal cholesterol levels - that occur together. These increase the risk of heart disease, stroke and diabetes. People on the Mediterranean diet have been found to be less likely to be overweight, thus reducing incidence of this condition.

A study showed that 13 thousand and 380 people who followed the Mediterranean diet, had a lower 83 per cent risk of diabetes type II, compared with those who did not bother using that system seriously. The research found that eating according to the Mediterranean diet leads to an improvement in cases of joint pain, and reduce the risk of pulmonary embolism, as well as reduce the risk of recurrence of colon cancer.

We do not know all the mechanisms that make a healthy Mediterranean diet completely, but research assumes the existence of a number of factors. And one reason only, the monounsaturated fat in olive oil and fish, have anti-inflammatory effects, which may help in the prevention of heart disease, and many other diseases.

The fiber in whole grains and legumes can help for digestion, and maintaining disciplined levels of blood sugar. The fiber also creates a feeling of fullness, a sense reduces the appetite - and this is one of the levers to reduce the increase in weight. The other elements in a vegetarian diet also have influences on the cellular level, and the aging process, the process of development of cancer, and the process of the body's response to chemotherapy.

Well, of course, eating according to the Mediterranean diet excludes many of the foods that are known to cause health problems such as saturated fat from animal sources, trans-fat and refined carbohydrates.

The Mediterranean diet has several advantages. The elements are already available, and can be prepared easily and quickly, the food varied and delicious taste. And dealt with after meals, it will not let you feel hungry or deprived. Use plenty of vegetables that almost are rich in nutrients and low in fat and calories. It is rich in fiber, and saturated with elements of health-promoting.

The key here is diversity; you must deal with different kinds. Instead of exposing them to steam or boil, try grilled or placed in the oven. Make salad a main dish for you, with the addition of nuts and small pieces of chicken or fish, and grated cheese. Eat plenty of fruits, vegetables, such as it is, a few in the caloric value of general and saturated nutrients, and antioxidants, and fiber.

Most fruits naturally have sweet taste, so it can serve as a snack or a great substitute for sweets and a meal. Type of fruit; definitely put them over the power. At breakfast in the morning you can eat whole grains or products with milk, yogurt and berries or pieces of banana. Eating nuts which contain a lot of antioxidants and other nutrients, For example, nuts contains «Omega-3» fatty acids, which reduce the risk of heart disease and blood vessels, and has adverse effects on the aging of the brain and skin.

Unlike the light products made from refined grains or mixed with refined sugar, the nuts have a function pointer a little sugar. However, the nuts are high in calories, so they fill up the hunger. Therefore, try not to deal with more than a handful of them (160 to 180 calories) per day. Sprinkle cooked vegetables from the veggie list with almonds. Dip fish or chicken with olive oil and crushed nuts, before grilling. Eat whole grains, which contain mostly carbohydrates that we need for energy consumption.

However, refined grains, such as white pasta, white rice, white bread, chips and products such as cornflakes and refined snacks, are virtually devoid of nutrients, including fiber cereal flakes. With little or no fiber therein, which slows digestion, the refined grain causes sudden increases in the blood sugar level.

Over time, this may lead to weight gain, heart disease and other disorders. Whole grains are rich in vitamins, minerals and proteins and have an influential role in the stability of the level of blood sugar. Perhaps you are now addressing bread from whole grains, brown rice, oats, but there are plenty of other delicious options.

Chapter Five

Mediterranean Diet & You

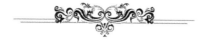

The Mediterranean diet is best for your heart. It is the way to eat and drink to your health. It is rich in vegetables, grains (rice, pasta), fish, fruit and dried beans.The Mediterranean diet is a wonderfully healthy diet and an extremely easy one to adapt to our stressful and fast paced lifestyles.

This diet is a balanced diet full of a variety of foods and can be followed easily. A main factor in the appeal is its rich, full flavored foods.It is also very low in saturated fat and includes plentiful amounts of fresh fruits and vegetables.

Another reason why the Mediterranean diet is good for you lies in the fact that the diet includes the consumption of a significant amount of fruit and vegetables.

Whether you want to lose weight, lower your cholesterol, eat more fruits and vegetables, or just feel healthier in general, adopting a Mediterranean diet is a great way to eat better while enjoying a delicious variety of food.

The Mediterranean diet is low in red meat and hence the diet plan works to reduce the amount of bad cholesterol.

The Mediterranean diet is high in whole grains and fiber as well as in anti-oxidants. It is also low in dairy products.

LONGEVITY

The history of the people of the Mediterranean region demonstrates that the Mediterranean diet works to extend a person's life.

The Mediterranean diet is one of the most suggested nutritional behaviors of the world. Adherence to it is associated with a significant reduction in mortality.Recent news reports that the Mediterranean diet is preferable for people suffering from diabetes over a low-carb diabetic diet.

There are a number of reasons why it is proving itself to be good for men of all ages. In addition to assisting men in fighting obesity and bringing their weight down to a healthy level, the Mediterranean diet is effective in aiding men to maintain a healthy weight over time.

In fact, the Mediterranean diet is simply closer to what people have eaten for millennia.

Numerous studies have shown that the low-fat, high-fiber Mediterranean diet is one of the best recipes against health problems such as arthritis, obesity, diabetes, asthma and cardiovascular disease.

In fact, the latest research now shows that Spain is at the top of the European longevity league tables and it is widely believed that the Mediterranean diet is responsible for this.The main oil used in the Mediterranean diet is olive, traditionally cold pressed virgin, and this is used not only for cooking and in salads, but also for putting on bread in place of butter.

Olive oil

Olive oil rather than butter or cream is the primary source of fat in Mediterranean diet. Olive oil is often used alone or in substitution for other oils, butter, and margarine.

It is rich in a type of fat that readily converts to a fatty acid similar to omega-3. Olive oil is used as the primary cooking oil in Italy and Greece, and is a source of monounsaturated fat, which is much easier for the body to break down.

Olive oil, produced from the olive trees prominent throughout Portugal, Greece, Croatia, Turkey, Italy, Spain and other Mediterranean nations, adds to the distinctive taste of the food.

Olive oil also offers several health advantages over more polyunsaturated vegetable oils. Olive oil compounds also increase enzymes that block activation of carcinogens and improve their removal from the body.

Olive oil is also a good source of antioxidants. It contains anti oxidant Oleic acid that reduces the risk of breast cancer. It also contains vitamins A, B1, B2, C, D, and K, and Iron Poli-phenols.

Olive oil has been associated with lower blood pressure, a lower risk for heart disease, and possible benefits for people with type 2 diabetes.

Foods are cooked with extra virgin olive oil and enjoyed with small amounts of red wine. Instead of cooking with butter and spreading it on foods, use olive oil or canola oil.

But unlike the saturated fats that we commonly eat (such as butter, margarine, vegetable oil, trans fats) the primary fats of the Mediterranean Diet consist of monounsaturated fats (found in Olive Oil) which provide the health benefits for your heart.

The research shows that wine is better than beer or spirits at protecting against heart disease, that olive oil can reduce the risk of bowel cancer and that garlic may lower cholesterol levels.

Vegetables

The Mediterranean diet is one that is rich in vegetables, grains (rice, pasta), fish, fruit and dried beans. The other important factor is to make the consumption of fruits and vegetables a daily habit.

The vitamins, minerals, photochemical and fiber provided by the diets large amounts of vegetables, fruits, grains and beans are believed to account for the inhabitants of the Mediterranean countries lower incidence of cancer otherwise commonly found in the United States.

The Mediterranean diet emphasizes intake of fruits and vegetables, whole grains, nuts, and legumes.

Substitute a changing array of fresh vegetables and legumes for rice and potato side dishes.

Fruits

Typical fruits consumed in Med diet are: apples, pears, oranges, Mandarin, apricots, peaches, grape, water-melons, melons, raspberries, strawberries, chestnuts, walnuts, nuts, almonds, and pistachio nuts.

People who follow the Mediterranean diet and consume generous servings of fruits and vegetables each day have a lower incidence of certain diseases, including cancer and cardiovascular ailments.

Nuts

Nuts, legumes, and beans are consumed daily.

Most of the studies have focused on the Mediterranean diet, emphasizing the consumption of high amounts of virgin / extra virgin olive oil (up to one liter per week) or nuts (up to 30 grams a day, or two handfuls), in comparison to a low-fat diet.

Foods like vegetables, nuts and monosaturated fatty acids are very beneficial for the heart.

But if you eat a reasonable amount of calories and swap out candy bars for nuts, the data says you will be healthier.

The Mediterranean diet shifts towards more plant-based nutrition, as well as proteins from sources like beans and nuts rather than red meats.

Some of the desirable food items:

Bread, pasta, rice,

Vegetables: Spinach, Cauliflowers, Carrots, Eggplants, Tomatoes, broccoli, capsicum, capers, garlic and onion

Fruit: Olives, Grape, Oranges, Lemons, Apples, cherries, Strawberries, peaches, apricots

Legumes: beans, peas

Nuts: Walnuts, Almonds, Pistachio nuts

Oil: olive

Honey

Milk and cheeses

White Meat (chicken, rabbit, turkey, etc...) and

Fish (fish sword, sardines, tuna, clears)

Eggs

Red meat (veal, lamb, etc...) (consume less)

Walnuts contain polyphenols and other anti-oxidants and essential fatty acids. Abundant vegetables, fiber-rich beans, fresh breads and healthy fats found in olives and nuts are the mainstay of this region and essential to everyone's good health and vitality.

The Mediterranean Diet is now recognized as one of the healthiest diets in the world.

REASONS WHY THE MEDITERRANEAN DIET IS GOOD FOR YOU

Low in Saturated Fat

Physicians and nutritionists the world over all agree that a diet that is high in saturated fat can have very negative consequences on a person's health and wellbeing. Indeed, a diet that is high in saturated fat can cause a person to suffer heart disease, can lead to cancer and can cause a whole host of other health problems and concern.

The Mediterranean diet is noteworthy because of the fact that it is very low in saturated fat. The typical person who follows the Mediterranean diet intakes less than eight percent of his or her calories from potentially harmful saturated fat. This is significantly below the average of people who do not follow a Mediterranean diet regimen.

Includes Plentiful Amounts of Fresh Fruits and Vegetables

Another reason why the Mediterranean diet is good for you lies in the fact that the diet includes the consumption of a significant amount of fruit and vegetables. Indeed, the diet encompasses more fresh fruits and vegetables than any other dietary program or plan today.

Fresh fruits and vegetables have a significant beneficial effect on a person's health and wellbeing. People who following the Mediterranean diet and consume generous servings of fruits and vegetables each day have a lower incidence of certain diseases including cancer and cardiovascular ailments.

High in Whole Grains and Fiber

A benefit in the Mediterranean diet is found in the fact that it lowers in the incidence of certain types of cancer. One of the reasons that the Mediterranean diet lowers the incidence of cancer is found in the fact that the diet is rich in whole grains and dietary fiber. Both whole grain and fiber have proven to lower the incidence of cancer, including colorectal cancer.

High in Anti-Oxidants

The Mediterranean diet is high in anti-oxidants. Anti-oxidants play a significant role in maintaining the body -- including organs, muscles and skin -- in top condition. A diet high in anti-oxidants is believed to ensure that a person will live a longer, healthier life.

Low in Red Meat

Because the Mediterranean diet is low in red meat, the diet plan works to reduce the amount of "bad cholesterol." A diet low in "bad cholesterol" lessens the incidence of cardiovascular disease, hypertension and stroke.

High in Lean Meats

The Mediterranean diet includes lean meats in moderate portions. The reasonable amount of lean meats --

including fish and certain seafood and fish -- provides a health source of protein and energy for a person.

Low in Dairy

The Mediterranean diet is low in dairy products. In fact, a true adherent to the Mediterranean diet includes almost no dairy products at all. Any dairy that is included in the diet is low fat or non-fat. Because the diet is low in dairy, particularly fatty dairy products, the diet encourages a person to obtain or maintain an ideal weight. Additionally, the diet aids in reducing cholesterol and works to prevent heart disease.

Prevents Disease

As mentioned, one of the reasons that the Mediterranean diet is good for you rests in the fact that the diet plan appears to reduce the incidence of certain diseases including:

- Heart and cardiovascular disease
- Cancer
- Diabetes
- Hypertension

- Diabetes

Longevity

The history of the people of the Mediterranean region demonstrates that the Mediterranean diet works to extend a person's life. In addition, while working to extend a person's life, this diet scheme works to ensure that a person's longer life will be healthy as well.

3 IMPORTANT EFFECTS OF THE MEDITERRANEAN DIET

Significant research studies have been undertaken since 1970 designed to isolate the benefits of the Mediterranean diet scheme. While the research into the possible benefits of the Mediterranean diet is ongoing and not yet complete, scientists, researchers and nutritionists from around the globe have concluded from their extensive research that the Mediterranean diet is beneficial on a number of levels:

1. Reducing the incidence of certain diseases
2. Increasing longevity
3. Providing for an overall healthier lifestyle

The Mediterranean Diet and Disease Risk Reduction

Over the course of the past thirty years, a significant amount of research has been undertaken to consider the possibility that the Mediterranean diet might be useful in lowering the incidence of certain types of diseases. A number of significant studies have been undertaken in this regard, including research that has included an analysis of the dining habits in people in different countries around the world over time.

These studies initially were motivated by the fact that the people who populate the region surrounding the Mediterranean Sea tended to have lower incidents of different types of serious diseases that are on the increase in many different countries around the world. In this regard, researchers wanted to determine whether the reason the people of the Mediterranean region seemed to enjoy better health was environmentally driven or the result of their particular diet regimens.

These studies have demonstrated that Mediterranean diet appears to be effective in lowering the incidence of certain types of diseases:

1. Cancer (including breast cancer and colorectal cancer)
2. Coronary Disease
3. Other Cardiovascular Disease
4. Hypertension

The Mediterranean Diet and Increased Longevity

Of course, it goes without saying that if a person is able to reduce the risks of certain diseases through his or her diet, that person has a far better chance of living a longer life. In addition, it has been demonstrated that the substantial benefits of the Mediterranean diet have a cumulative effect on and for the human body.

What this means is that the longer a person follows the dining practices of the peoples of the Mediterranean region, the more ingrained the benefits of the diet become within the body. In simple terms, by utilizing and practicing the Mediterranean diet over time, a person will enjoy lasting benefits that will prolong his or her life.

By way of example, one might consider the negative consequences of smoking. If you elect to smoke cigarettes over a long period of time, you will cause irreparable harm to your body. Conversely, if you diligently follow the guidelines of the Mediterranean diet over time, your body will enjoy definitive and lasting benefits that will include good health and a longer life.

The Mediterranean Diet and Your General Health

Research has demonstrated that people who follow the Mediterranean diet are afflicted with fewer minor ailments such as colds and the flu than are their counterparts who follow other types of dining routines. In short, and on many levels, research over the course of three decades that people who follow a Mediterranean diet are afflicted with fewer illnesses, have more energy and suffer from the effects of being overweight or obese far less often than people who utilized other dietary practices.

WHY THE MEDITERRANEAN DIET IS GOOD FOR WOMEN

Over the course of the past forty years, women the world over have become particularly concerned about their diets. They have become concerned about diet related issues for two primary reasons:

1. Women have expressed concern over how a particular diet plan effects their appearances

2. Women have expressed concern over how a particular dies plan effects their health

As a result, a growing number of women have found themselves attracted to the Mediterranean diet. When it comes to the Mediterranean diet, there are six primary reasons why women find themselves strongly attracted to the diet regimen.

3. Weight Loss and Healthy Weight Maintenance

In many countries around the world, a record number of women are being classified as overweight and even obese. As a result, a growing number of women find themselves seeking effective and healthy dieting regimens to lower their weight to appropriate levels -- for both cosmetic as well as health reasons.

The Mediterranean diet has proven itself to be very effective at providing a means through which women can lose weight in a healthy manner. Additionally, the Mediterranean diet has proven incredibly effective as being a solid path a woman can take to maintain a generally ideal and healthy weight.

4. Anti-oxidants and Aging

The Mediterranean diet regimen is flush with foods that are rich in anti-oxidants. This includes leafy, dark green vegetables as well as certain fish that are common features in this dietary scheme.

Anti-oxidants have been proven to slow the appearance of aging in women. Additionally, anti-oxidants have been demonstrated as being effective at preventing organ and skin deterioration in women. The consumption of foods that are high in anti-oxidants has been proven to enhance longevity in both women and men.

5.Metabolic Syndrome

Metabolic syndrome is an ailment in which a person ends up afflicted with both Type Two diabetes and hypertension. Most experts believe that diet can play a significant role in reducing the likelihood of metabolic syndrome in men and women who are prone to the ailment.

Without exception, medical experts who have studied the cause and effect of metabolic syndrome universally have agreed that the Mediterranean diet is the perfect dietary scheme to prevent and control metabolic syndrome.

6. Heart Disease

Multiple studies in a number of different countries have concluded that the adoption of the Mediterranean diet lowers the incidence of heart disease in women (and men). Indeed, an analysis of the incidence of heart disease in the Mediterranean nations suggests that the use of the Mediterranean diet can lower the incidence of heart disease in women from twenty-five to forty percent.

7. Hypertension

Recent scientific studies have examined the rising incidence of hypertension amongst women. Many researchers attribute the increase in hypertension amongst women in recent years to a number of changes that have occurred in their lives, including:

- A greater number of women entering the workforce
- A growing number of women being forced to juggle the raising of children with a full-time career
- The food and beverage choices that women are making in the 21st century

Research studies in a dozen different countries over the course of the past twenty years have suggested that the Mediterranean diet is effective at lowering the incidence of hypertension in men and women. Because the Mediterranean diet is high if fruit, vegetables and whole grains and because the diet is low in saturated fats, most nutritionists and other experts believe that the dietary scheme works to lower hypertension in both men and women.

The Mediterranean diet combined with regular exercise has been demonstrated to have a marked effect on reducing the incidence of hypertension amongst middle-aged women.

8. Breast Cancer

Perhaps the most important "ingredient" of the Mediterranean diet is olive oil. Save for fresh fruits and vegetables (in most instances) olive oil universally is present in the Mediterranean diet. As a result, on the surface, the diet scheme appears to be high in fat. Indeed, upwards to thirty percent of the caloric intake of the Mediterranean diet does come fat. What is important to keep in mind is that nearly 100% of the fat in the Mediterranean diet is unsaturated and comes directly from olive oil. In other words, the fat in the Mediterranean diet essentially is healthy. Olive oil, and the fat contained in the product, simply does not trigger the negative consequences that flow from saturated fats, from animal fats.

In addition, there have been several important scientific studies undertaken in the past decade that have demonstrated that a diet high in olive oil works to lower the risk of breast cancer in women. Thus, one of the beneficial results of adopting the Mediterranean diet is a lowering of the risk for breast cancer.

THE MEDITERRANEAN DIET IS GOOD FOR MEN

One of the primary concerns of a growing number of men the world over is finding a diet and exercise plan that will assist in ensuring that they are in optimal health. In recent years, a significant number of men have found themselves attracted to the Mediterranean diet. These men have come to learn that the Mediterranean is a solid choice for assisting them in developing a comprehensive regimen for health living.

There are a number of reasons why the Mediterranean diet is proving itself to be good for men of all ages.

1. The Mediterranean Diet Reduces the Risks of Some Serious Diseases

Over the course of the past thirty years, a number of research studies have been conducted pertaining to the Mediterranean diet regimen. These studies have produced results that demonstrate that the Mediterranean diet can prove effective in reducing the incidence of a number of serious diseases and ailments in men.

The diseases in men that the Mediterranean diet appears to help prevent include:

- Cancer
- Heart and cardiovascular disease
- Hypertension
- Gallstones
- Stroke
- Diabetes

2. The Mediterranean Diet is Effective in Helping Men Reach and Keep an Ideal Weight

Many men are confronting problems related with being overweight and obesity. Indeed, in some countries, obesity is becoming the number one health concern amongst men of all ages.

Because the Mediterranean diet includes the consumption of generous portions of fresh fruits and vegetables, whole grains and lean meats, the diet can be very effective in assisting a man in bringing his weight down to a healthy, ideal level.

In addition to assisting men in fighting obesity and bringing their weight down to a healthy level, the Mediterranean diet is effective in aiding men to maintain a healthy weight over time. While it is one thing for a person to be able to lose weight, it is a completely different challenge for a man to be able to keep weight off over the long term. The Mediterranean diet has proven itself time and again as being a solid dietary program through which a person can maintain a healthy weight.

3. The Mediterranean Diet -- Adding Years to a Man's Life

Throughout history, the males who have populated the region in and around the Mediterranean Sea have been found to live lives longer than their counterparts in other parts of the world. In time, experts in the field of nutrition were able to demonstrate that men in the Mediterranean region lived longer because of their diets.

Scientists and other researchers have been able to demonstrate that there are positive, cumulative effects associated with the Mediterranean diet. In other words, by utilizing and following the Mediterranean diet over time, a man's life (in many instances) will be extended. In addition to having the chance to live a longer life because of dietary decisions, a man's life will be healthier and more robust because of his adherence to the Mediterranean diet scheme.

Chapter Six

Longevity And The Mediterranean Diet

Over the course of many generations, observers have been able to discern that the people who populate the region around the Mediterranean Sea live longer lives than do men and women in some other parts of the world. Historically, the reason most often attributed to the longevity of the people of the Mediterranean region was climate.

However, as researchers became more adept and as scientific methods became more sophisticated, it became clear that while the weather patterns of the Mediterranean area generally were pleasant and inviting, it was the diet of the people in the region that accounted for their longer lives.

There are a number of specific factors related to the Mediterranean diet that nutritionists and medical experts believe contribute to longevity. The more important of these elements are discussed within the confines of this article for your information and guidance.

1. Restorative Effects of the Mediterranean Diet

Many of the specific food items that are part of a Mediterranean diet regimen are high in anti-oxidants. Scientifically speaking, anti-oxidants are important compounds found in certain foods and beverages that work to neutralize the destructive nature of oxidants or free radicals that are found in the human body. Oxidants or free radicals are produced when the body burns oxygen to produce energy. In other words, oxidants really can be considered waste that pollutes the human body.

Over time, the accumulation of oxidants in the body accelerates the aging process. Cells wear and lose their elasticity. Organs end up functioning less efficiently and effectively. Indeed, recent scientific research has demonstrated that oxidants clog arteries raising the threat of stroke. Oxidants are found to contribute to cancer, heart disease and diabetes -- the major diseases most responsible for causing people to have premature deaths.

The types of fruits and vegetables that form the foundation of the Mediterranean diet -- including richly colored and leafy green vegetables -- which are high in anti-oxidants, have a restorative and life prolonging effect on the typical human body.

2. Reducing Cancer Risks

In most parts of the world, cancer of various types is the leading cause of premature death. Studies undertaken by researchers in Europe, Japan and the United States in the past thirty years have demonstrated that the Mediterranean diet effectively reduces the risks of certain types of cancers.

A diet that is high in fresh fruits and vegetables has been shown to be effective in reducing the risks of a wide array of different types of cancers. As has been noted previously, the Mediterranean diet includes the generous consumption of fresh fruits and vegetables.

The Mediterranean diet includes very little animal fat. There is a direct link between the consumption of animal fat and colorectal cancer, one of the deadliest forms of the disease that oftentimes takes the lives of people in their forties and fifties.

Olive oil (truly the foundation of the Mediterranean diet) had been shown to reduce the risk of breast cancer.

By reducing the risks poised by cancer, the lifespan of men and women has been shown to increase appreciably in studies that have followed groups of people over time.

3. Reducing Coronary Heart Disease Risks

Coronary heart disease is one of the top three causes of premature death throughout the world -- except in the Mediterranean region. Researchers have concluded that diet has played a large and important role in reducing the risk of coronary heart disease amongst the people who populate the countries surrounding the Mediterranean Sea.

An important study in seven countries (Italy, Greece, Yugoslavia, Finland, United States, Netherlands and Japan) demonstrated that those people who followed a Mediterranean diet regimen were less likely to have coronary heart disease and were less likely to have their lives cut short because of serious and ultimately fatal heart conditions.

4. Reducing Hypertension

On some level, the jury is still out on the direct effects between diet and hypertension or high blood pressure. With that said, it clearly has been demonstrated that hypertension and high blood pressure is responsible for premature deaths the world over. In addition, there is strong evidence to suggest that eliminating certain items from a diet -- like processed salts -- can work to reduce the risk of hypertension.

Additionally, there is evidence to support the proposition that a diet high in fiber and low in animal fats (like that of the Mediterranean region) works to reduce the threat of hypertension and premature death from this disease.

5. Diabetes Prevention and Control

The Mediterranean diet is well suited to staving off the serious effects of diabetes. The incidence of premature death because of diabetes is lower in those regions in which the Mediterranean diet is practiced. Because diabetes is a disease that can be controlled through diet, electing to utilize the Mediterranean regimen can work to add literally years to a person's life.

6. The Cumulative Effect of the Mediterranean Diet

It is important to note that the beneficial effects of the Mediterranean diet appear to be cumulative over time. In the other words, the longer a person practices the dining habits of the Mediterranean plan, more of inherent physical benefits of this healthy eating regimen will be ingrained into a person's makeup. Simply put, the benefits of a Mediterranean diet literally are stored up over time, increasing a person's lifespan and adding to his or her overall health and wellbeing not only now, but well into the future.

Mediterranean Diet-Ways to Living a Longer,Without Heart Disease

1. Watch what type of fuel you feed your body

Why do many people buy Super gasoline even though it's more expensive? If they bought the least expensive gas they could save a lot of money. Well, only in the short run. Car engines run more efficiently with high-quality fuels and the parts deteriorate much faster when you use cheap fluids.

Like your car, your body is comprised of different parts and your heart is the engine. The fuel you use to keep your heart and other body parts running makes a difference in your performance, whether you're at work, at school, with your family or anywhere else. It will also affect the speed at which your parts deteriorate.

Nowadays, nutrition experts all over the world are making an effort to introduce the principles of the Mediterranean diet because centuries of experience have proved that it is the best "fuel" available to keep our "parts" running well until old age. Even the European community is recommending this healthy diet to all its members.

2. Cut down on processed foods and load up with fruits and vegetables

To have a healthy heart like the Mediterraneans and maintain normal blood pressure, your diet should be five times higher in potassium than in sodium -the part of salt that is bad for us. Unfortunately, in the typical American diet, the amount of sodium is five times higher than potassium. Why do we have it so backwards? Because seventy-five percent of the salt we eat every day comes from processed foods, most of which is added by manufacturers and restaurants.

Because the American public consumes about 4,000mg per day of sodium, far more than what is needed, the American Public Health Association recently called for a 50 percent sodium reduction in our nation's food supply over the next ten years. It's estimated that such a reduction would save at least 150,000 lives annually.

Fruits and vegetables are low in sodium and high in potassium. By eating fruits and vegetables, you are also replacing other foods in your meals that may be high in sodium. Plus fruits and vegetables contribute good amounts of calcium and magnesium, two minerals that you need for a normal heartrate and to maintain low blood pressure.

3. Give yourself a daily dose of olive oil

Replace saturated fat with extra virgin olive oil. Butter is rarely consumed in the traditional Mediterranean diet and margarine was completely unknown in the area until recently. People in the Mediterranean countries use extra virgin olive oil, one of the best sources of monounsaturated fat, the kind of fat that does not stick to your arteries. Extra virgin olive oil is also an excellent source of many antioxidants such as vitamin E.

If you are considering taking vitamin E in capsules, be aware that you won't get the same results as ingesting extra virgin olive oil. Researchers for the Heart Outcomes Prevention Evaluation Study found that people who received 265 milligrams of vitamin E daily in the form of supplements did not have fewer hospitalizations for heart failure or chest pain when compared to those who received a placebo, a faked pill. That's why nutrition authorities recommend 2 to 3 tablespoons of extra virgin olive oil a day as prevention. So use olive oil and avoid other fat sources such as butter and margarine.

4. Eat more legumes

By legumes, I mean dry beans, lentils, chickpeas and garbanzo beans. Legumes have been a staple food in the Mediterranean diet for centuries. They are packed with minerals such as iron, magnesium, manganese, phosphorous, zinc, potassium, folic acid and some of the B-complex vitamins. They are low in fat and sodium. Legumes are also very high in soluble fiber, which takes cholesterol out of your body through the feces. And to top it all, legumes can help balance your budget because they are very inexpensive. If legumes are not part of your regular diet, you are missing an almost perfect food.

5. Eat more aromatic herbs, garlic and onions

To add the Mediterranean flavor to your meals, replace salt with garlic and aromatic herbs. Garlic is a truly wonder of nature; it has been used for thousands of years as both food and medicine. People around the world, especially those who enjoy fewer chronic heart diseases, use it extensively in their daily diets. Why? Because more than 200 chemical compounds that might protect our bodies have been found in garlic.

Recent studies have shown that garlic can significantly reduce cholesterol and triglycerides, lower blood pressure and prevent the formation of blood clots. It can also protect our bodies through its antioxidant properties.

Onions and other aromatic herbs work very similar to garlic. They contain about 25 active compounds that appear to help combat heart disease, strokes, high blood pressure and cholesterol.

Chapter Seven

Mediterranean Diet Planners

The Mediterranean diet comprises of foods such as cereals, grains, vegetables, dried beans, olive oil, garlic, fresh herbs, seafood, and fruits. Mediterranean diet planners are the nutritionists or dieticians who recommend people with health problems follow a Mediterranean diet.

They plan a specific diet for people with faulty eating habits that can culminate in obesity and other ailments. They focus upon a diet rich in fiber. This intake is naturally contained in fresh herbs, seafood, and fruits and vegetables. People are encouraged to follow a modified Mediterranean diet in which unsaturated fats are substituted with monounsaturated fats, as there is evidence that these ensure longer life expectancy.

Mediterranean diet planners highlight the importance of using olive oil as a cooking medium and dressings for salads. They plan meals that include moderate amounts of fish and meat and low to moderate amounts of cheese and yogurt. They focus on a meal rich in the consumption of fruits, vegetables, potatoes, beans, nuts, seeds, bread and other cereals. The meals also include consumption of wine in moderation.

The diet planners gain information from their patients, before formulating a Mediterranean diet plan for an individual. They acknowledge personal tastes and preferences when they plan a diet for a week or a month. They also make changes in the daily menu, which ensures that the patients are not deprived of their favorite foods and enjoy their daily Mediterranean cuisine with relish.

The planners do not advice people to strictly adhere to the Mediterranean diet but to enjoy a change that rejuvenates their health.

CHOOSE THE RIGHT DIET PLAN - MEDITERRANEAN DIET REVIEW

Choosing Heart-Healthy Options with the Mediterranean Diet

There are many diets out there you can choose from, but for many the Mediterranean diet will be one of the best choices. This is a very healthy diet that can help those with heart issues, high cholesterol, or other health problems. It is an eating plan that will help you discover how to create great tasting meals that are also very good for your heart.

This may be the only diet that includes drinking a glass of red wine, but that has been proven to be very good for your heart. The Mediterranean diet is based around the typical cooking styles of the countries on the coast of the Mediterranean Sea. They love to use olive oil in their cooking, so you can expect to get plenty of good meals made with the health benefits of olive oil.

When you are trying to diet because of the risk of heart disease, it is not as good to use a traditional diet. Even though the same parts, like eating plenty of fruits and vegetables, fish, and whole grains are the same, the Mediterranean Diet helps you take it one step further by giving you the right proportions of the right foods for your heart.

Many studies have been done and they have proven that the traditional Mediterranean Diet will help to reduce the risk of heart disease. This type of diet has also been linked to reduction in cancer, and a reduction in the incidence of Parkinson's and Alzheimer's disease. It is all about good foods cooked in the right ways to keep your heart healthy.

What Does the Mediterranean Diet Emphasize?

There are many things included within the Mediterranean Diet and you need to be aware of what you are getting into. The key components, just like any other diet, are proper eating habits and exercise. In fact, the Mediterranean Diet puts a strong emphasis on getting plenty of exercise each week because this makes a huge difference in heart health.

The Mediterranean Diet also includes eating mainly plant-based foods like vegetables, fruits, legumes, nuts, and whole grains. This does not mean you are a vegetarian on this diet, but you will not be eating as much meat as you may be used to. This diet only calls for eating red meat a few times a month and fish and poultry at least twice a week.

You will also be replacing butter with healthy fats like canola oil and olive oil with this diet. This will help to give your body the fat it needs, but only in the right forms instead of in the bad fats like butter contains. Another big part of the Mediterranean Diet is using herbs and spices instead of salt to flavor your foods.

There is one last component to the Mediterranean Diet and it is the best one of all. It is, of course, optional, but a very large part of the culture of this area of the world and one that many people love. You are supposed to drink red wine in moderation when on the Mediterranean Diet because it is proven a glass of wine with dinner is good for your heart and your body.

Another important part of the diet is enjoying meals with your family and your friends. This is a tradition in the Mediterranean culture and it goes along with the diet. Every component is added because it gives the body the necessary nutrients and it is also very healthy for the heart. This is one of the best diets for anybody with a history of heart disease or high cholesterol.

What I Think About the Mediterranean Diet

Whether you are looking for a healthier way to live and eat or you are looking for a diet to help you lose weight, the Mediterranean Diet is a good choice. You are not going to drop 20 pounds in a month with this diet, but it will help you get to a very healthy weight and maintain it. This is not just a diet you start and finish, but also a way of changing the way you eat every single day for the rest of your life.

It is nice to find a diet that does not completely cut out the things you may enjoy. You can still have red meat, just not that often and you are even encouraged to drink wine with this diet. Most diets do not allow any alcohol and will cut out many of the things you really need. With the Mediterranean Diet, you can have confidence in knowing that you are eating in a hearth healthy way that supports the body completely.

Chapter Eight

Mediterranean Diet Recipes

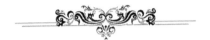

1. FETA GARBANZO BEAN SALAD

INGREDIENTS

- 1 can (15 ounces) garbanzo beans, rinsed and drained
- 1-1/2 cups coarsely chopped English cucumber (about 1/2 medium)
- 1 can (2-1/4 ounces) sliced ripe olives, drained
- 1 medium tomato, seeded and chopped
- 1/4 cup thinly sliced red onion
- 1/4 cup chopped fresh parsley
- 3 tablespoons olive oil
- 1 tablespoon lemon juice
- 1/4 teaspoon salt

- 1/8 teaspoon pepper
- 5 cups torn mixed salad greens
- 1/2 cup crumbled feta cheese

Total Time

- Prep/Total Time: 15 min.
- Makes
- 4 servings

Directions

Place the first 11 ingredients in a large bowl; toss to combine. Sprinkle with cheese.

Nutrition Facts

2 cups: 268 calories, 16g fat (3g saturated fat), 8mg cholesterol, 586mg sodium, 24g carbohydrate (4g sugars, 7g fiber), 9g protein.

2. COD AND ASPARAGUS BAKE

Ingredients

- 4 cod fillets (4 ounces each)

- 1 pound fresh thin asparagus, trimmed
- 1 pint cherry tomatoes, halved
- 2 tablespoons lemon juice
- 1-1/2 teaspoons grated lemon zest
- 1/4 cup grated Romano cheese

Total Time

- Prep/Total Time: 30 min.
- Makes
- 4 servings

Directions

Preheat oven to 375°. Place cod and asparagus in a 15x10x1-in. baking pan brushed with oil. Add tomatoes, cut side down. Brush fish with lemon juice; sprinkle with lemon zest. Sprinkle fish and vegetables with Romano cheese. Bake until fish just begins to flake easily with a fork, about 12 minutes.

Remove pan from oven; preheat broiler. Broil cod mixture 3-4 in. from heat until vegetables are lightly browned, 2-3 minutes.

Nutrition Facts

1 serving: 141 calories, 3g fat (2g saturated fat), 45mg cholesterol, 184mg sodium, 6g carbohydrate (3g sugars, 2g fiber), 23g protein.

3. SALMON WITH SPINACH & WHITE BEANS

Ingredients

- 4 salmon fillets (4 ounces each)
- 2 teaspoons plus 1 tablespoon olive oil, divided
- 1 teaspoon seafood seasoning
- 1 garlic clove, minced
- 1 can (15 ounces) cannellini beans, rinsed and drained
- 1/4 teaspoon salt
- 1/4 teaspoon pepper
- 1 package (8 ounces) fresh spinach
- Lemon wedges

Total Time

- Prep/Total Time: 15 min.
- Makes

- 4 servings

Directions

Preheat broiler. Rub fillets with 2 teaspoons oil; sprinkle with seafood seasoning. Place on a greased rack of a broiler pan. Broil 5-6 in. from heat 6-8 minutes or until fish just begins to flake easily with a fork.

Meanwhile, in a large skillet, heat remaining oil over medium heat. Add garlic; cook 15-30 seconds or until fragrant. Add beans, salt and pepper, stirring to coat beans with garlic oil. Stir in spinach until wilted. Serve salmon with spinach mixture and lemon wedges.

Nutrition Facts

1 fillet with 1/2 cup spinach mixture : 317 calories, 17g fat (3g saturated fat), 57mg cholesterol, 577mg sodium, 16g carbohydrate (0 sugars, 5g fiber), 24g protein.

4. SKILLET CHICKEN WITH OLIVES

Ingredients

- 4 boneless skinless chicken thighs (about 1 pound)
- 1 teaspoon dried rosemary, crushed
- 1/2 teaspoon pepper
- 1/4 teaspoon salt
- 1 tablespoon olive oil
- 1/2 cup pimiento-stuffed olives, coarsely chopped
- 1/4 cup white wine or chicken broth
- 1 tablespoon drained capers, optional

Total Time

- Prep/Total Time: 20 min.
- Makes
- 4 servings

Directions

Sprinkle chicken with rosemary, pepper and salt. In a large skillet, heat oil over medium-high heat. Brown chicken on both sides.

Add olives, wine and, if desired, capers. Reduce heat; simmer, covered, 2-3 minutes or until a thermometer inserted in chicken reads 170°.

Nutrition Facts

1 serving (calculated without capers): 237 calories, 15g fat (3g saturated fat), 76mg cholesterol, 571mg sodium, 2g carbohydrate (0 sugars, 0 fiber), 21g protein.

5. MEDITERRANEAN PORK AND ORZO

Ingredients

- 1-1/2 pounds pork tenderloin
- 1 teaspoon coarsely ground pepper
- 2 tablespoons olive oil
- 3 quarts water
- 1-1/4 cups uncooked orzo pasta
- 1/4 teaspoon salt
- 1 package (6 ounces) fresh baby spinach
- 1 cup grape tomatoes, halved
- 3/4 cup crumbled feta cheese

Total Time

- Prep/Total Time: 30 min.
- Makes
- 6 servings

Directions

Rub pork with pepper; cut into 1-in. cubes. In a large nonstick skillet, heat oil over medium heat. Add pork; cook and stir 8-10 minutes or until no longer pink.

Meanwhile, in a Dutch oven, bring water to a boil. Stir in orzo and salt; cook, uncovered, 8 minutes. Stir in spinach; cook 45-60 seconds longer or until orzo is tender and spinach is wilted. Drain.

Add tomatoes to pork; heat through. Stir in orzo mixture and cheese.

Nutrition Facts

1-1/3 cups: 372 calories, 11g fat (4g saturated fat), 71mg cholesterol, 306mg sodium, 34g carbohydrate (2g sugars, 3g fiber), 31g protein.

6. GRILLED SQUID

Ingredients

- 800 gr squid
- 2 lemon
- pepper q.s.

- 2 clove garlic
- extra virgin olive oil 1dl
- 50 gr parsley
- Salt to taste

Total Time

- Prep/Total Time: 15 min.
- Makes
- 4 servings

Directions

1) Clean the squid by separating the heads from the body, wash and dry them.

2) Season with salt and a drizzle of oil, cook them on a very hot grill turning them on one side and on the other.

3) Emulsify salt, pepper, parsley and garlic finely chopped with a small glass of oil.

4) Place the squid in a hot dish, season with the sauce and serve with the lemons cut into quarters.

Nutrition facts

Per 100g : 171 calories, 12gr Fat, 3gr carbohydrates, 13gr protein, 71gr water

7. SPAGHETTI OIL, GARLIC AND CHILLI

Ingredients:

- 320gr spaghetti
- garlic 3 cloves
- oil 70gr
- chili pepper 3

Total time

- Prep/Total Time 15 min.
- Makes
- 4 servings

Directions

To prepare spaghetti, garlic, oil and chilli, start by cooking the pasta in boiling salted water to taste.

Cook the spaghetti al dente and in the meantime you can prepare the sauce: peel the garlic cloves, cut them in half and remove the soul (the central green part of each clove).

Reduce the slices into rather thin slices. Take the fresh chilli, and cut it into slices eliminating the stalk. If you prefer a smaller spiciness, you can open it for the sense of length and remove the seeds before reducing it to slices. Now pour the oil into a large pan.

Heat it over a low heat and add the garlic and chilli. Fry the sauce on a very low flame, chilli and garlic will not burn but just fry for a couple of minutes and for a uniform browning without the risk of burning them, you can tilt the pan to collect oil and seasoning in a single point and allow uniform browning. Once the pasta is cooked al dente, you can transfer it directly to the pan and add a ladle of cooking water.

Stir a few moments to mix the flavors and sauté everything, then you can serve your spaghetti with garlic oil and chilli to serve it hot!

Nutrition facts:

for 80gr: Calories 388 kcal, Protein 8.8 g, Carbohydrates 66.4 g, Fat 11.5 g

Conclusions

During the past twenty years, a significant number of people in different countries around the world have turned their attention towards finding healthy diet regimens that are low in saturated fat and that include bountiful servings of fresh fruits and vegetable.

Consequently, the Mediterranean diet has caught the eye of innumerable people who want to include healthy eating into their overall course of prudent living. In short, the Mediterranean diet encompasses foods and beverages that, when consumed in moderation, can work to lessen the threat of some serious diseases and can aid in creating the necessary foundation for a long, hearty lifetime.

The Mediterranean diet is not just a way to lose weight, but is a way to entirely change your life, and in doing so, helping to prolong it. The health benefits are endless, especially when they are combined with exercise, making this nutrition adventure something definitely worth looking into.

Anti-inflammatory diet for beginners

The complete guide to reducing inflammation in our body, preventing or treating the resulting diseases and living a healthy life

GILLIAN WILLET

will any legal responsibility or blame be held against the publisher for any reparation, damages, or monetary loss due to the information herein, either directly or indirectly.

Respective authors own all copyrights not held by the publisher.

The information herein is offered for informational purposes solely, and is universal as so. The presentation of the information is without contract or any type of guarantee assurance.

The trademarks that are used are without any consent, and the publication of the trademark is without permission or backing by the trademark owner. All trademarks and brands within this book are for clarifying purposes only and are the owned by the owners themselves, not affiliated with this document

Table of Contents

Introduction

With so much pollution, tension and stress taking their toll on our health, the one thing that we can do to battle this is to have a nutrition rich anti inflammation diet.

Pollution causes free radical damage and also has serious inflammatory effects which have tremendous adverse effects on our health, leading to numerous ailments including psoriasis, cancer, auto immune diseases, Alzheimer's disease, heart diseases etc. Can an anti-inflammation diet help here?

Of course it can. In fact that is one of the best ways to come out victorious from this maze of diseases and disorders. An anti-inflammation diet should strictly consist of omega 3 fatty acids which have amazing anti-inflammatory properties. These fatty acids are essentially comprised of DHA (Docosahexanoic Acid) and EPA (Eicosapentaenoic Acid) fats.

Our body internally converts DHA into a substance called Resolvin D2 which is a potent and effective anti-inflammatory agent. It works by inhibiting the production of pro-inflammatory eicosanoids which reduce the inflammation significantly and provide instant relief from various ailments including the common ones like arthritis and gout.

If you want to make this beneficial fatty acid a part of your daily diet, one best and efficient way is to incorporate premium fish oil supplements in your health regimen. Make sure to choose the one having more DHA content than EPA.

This not only helps in ensuring the anti-inflammatory properties contained in DHA but also ensures ample supply of both DHA and EPA to the body. This is due to our body's ability to convert DHA into EPA as per its requirement. Since the reverse reaction is difficult to attain, it is advisable to take a supplement containing more DHA content.

These supplements not only regularize and assure your receiving an anti-inflammation diet, it also ensures that you take it in optimal amounts. The good supplements have the optimal usage per serving specified on them which is one thing to be checked before choosing to incorporate them in your daily regimen.

This complete guide is fully packed with tons of information about both an anti-inflammation diet as well as how to incorporate it in your routine, I hope you are going to take it forward and put it to the test right away. Take the decision and take it soon, after all there is nothing better than enjoying good health for years to come.

Happy Reading.

Chapter 1

The Anti-Inflammatory Diet

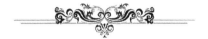

Chronic inflammation is a type of inflammation that silently attacks the body causing disease and degeneration, and is also known as "silent inflammation". As the connection between silent inflammation and a host of diseases becomes clearer, the case for dietary and lifestyle changes that can combat inflammation has become stronger.

While it was always known that some conditions such as arthritis and acne were a result of acute inflammation in the body, there is mounting evidence that silent inflammation plays a role in heart disease, Alzheimer's, diabetes and some cancers, as well as in the ageing process. Chronic inflammation can be present undetected in your body for years, until it manifests in disease.

Silent inflammation has been linked with the buildup of cholesterol deposits in the arteries which can lead to heart disease. In a similar way, the risk of Alzheimer's disease increases with inflammation of brain tissue, as this results in the buildup of amyloid plaque deposits in the brain.

Having type 2 diabetes, or eating sugary foods contributes to silent inflammation in the body as a result of elevated blood sugar and insulin levels. Recent studies have also confirmed the link between inflammation and several types of cancers. Making the necessary lifestyle changes to fight inflammation, can protect you from its devastating effects.

There are molecules in the body called prostaglandins which play an important role in inflammation. It has been found that of the three main types of prostaglandins, two of them (PG-E1 and PG-E3) have an anti-inflammatory effect, while the third type (PG-E2) actually promotes inflammation. When there is an imbalance in the body between these prostaglandins, inflammation can result.

Prostaglandins are made in the body from essential fatty acids. You can assist your body in making anti-Inflammatory prostaglandins by eating vegetables, nuts, grains and seeds such as sesame and sunflower seeds.

On the other hand, foods that cause a spike in insulin levels, such as sugary foods, or foods with a high Glycemic load promote production of PG-E2 and increase inflammation.

A typical anti-inflammatory diet focuses on fighting inflammation through the consumption of foods that lower insulin levels.

To actively reduce inflammation, you should therefore eat foods that have a low Glycemic load, such as whole grains, vegetables and lentils, and consume healthy fats such as nuts, seeds, fish, extra virgin olive oil and fish. Spices such as turmeric, ginger, and hot peppers also reduce inflammation.

At the same time, you also need to reduce consumption of foods that are pro-inflammatory, such as red meat, egg yolks and shellfish.

Sugar is a key culprit in inflammation, and therefore you should also cut back on sugary foods. Inflammation can also be reduced by taking supplements such as fish oils which are high in Omega 3 fatty acids.

Chapter 2

The Benefits Of An Anti-Inflammatory Diet

People suffering from obesity have inflammation issues. Diabetes, arthritis and asthma are all associated with inflammation in the body. Not to mention the link to certain heart conditions and cancers.

Reducing the inflammation in your body with an anti-inflammation diet can cause an immediate change to how you feel, not to mention the long term effects of the dietary change on health and well-being.

The first step to adopting an anti-inflammatory diet is to understand the effects of foods on the body. Food provides nutrients and vitamins the body needs to survive. The idea of eating to live not living to eat is a huge push for the weight loss community, but this idea should not just be followed when needing to lose a few pounds.

Certain foods have high concentrations of anti-oxidants and natural anti-inflammatory nutrients that may reduce the effect of inflammation on the body. It is these foods that cornerstone the anti-inflammatory diet.

The Role of Omega 3 and Other Fatty Acids

Fatty acids are present in many foods that contain oil. The best natural source is fish like salmon and sardines. However, Omega 6 fatty acids are prevalent in western diets over Omega 3s. This is because common eaten foods like chicken, turkey, eggs, nuts and vegetable oils are rich in Omega 6 fatty acids.

What people don't realize, however, is that these fatty acids need to be balanced with Omega 3s for optimal health and anti-inflammatory action. Most western diets include 10 times more Omega 6s than Omega 3s. Some diets include as much as 30 times more. The optimal ratio is 4 parts Omega 6 to every 1 part Omega 3.

Increasing Omega 3 fatty acids in the diet can reduce inflammation in the body and thus reduce the effect of this condition on health and general well-being. Foods rich in Omega 3s include fish oil, kiwi, black raspberry and various nuts.

The most readily available source of Omega 3s is flaxseeds. Many people mistake fish oils for the best source, but flaxseed oils tend to have the most readily available Omega 3s that make absorption in the body easier. Flaxseed oils contain about 55% ALA (alpha-linoleic acid) which is an Omega 3 fatty acid.

Another simple change to reduce inflammation in the body is the reduction of fatty meats. Red meat is the worst of all meats for people suffering from inflammation. Choosing a leaner cut or a leaner alternative is a good option. Bison and venison are two options that tend to contain less fat.

Grass fed cows also have fewer inflammatory characteristics on the body. Fish, lean chicken, turkey, soybeans, tofu and soy milk are all lean choices for decreasing inflammation. But some of these meats tend to be higher in Omega 6s.

To combat the fatty acid imbalance that may be increasing inflammation, try cooking these meats in olive oil or adding flaxseed oil to the final dish to boost Omega 3s.

The Danger of Processed Foods

The worst food to eat when suffering from inflammation is a processed carbohydrate. These foods offer very little nutritional value and should be replaced with whole grain alternatives. All flour is wheat based, but processed flour is stripped of the healthy grain wholeness and bleached.

What are left are empty calories sure to swell the body even more. Simply replacing white bread with whole grain bread and white flour with whole wheat flour that is unbleached can make a big difference in how your body reacts to your diet.

Chapter 3

Eating Anti-Inflammatory Foods

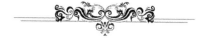

Scientists have found that there is a relationship, in part, between what we eat and inflammation. They've even identified some compounds in food that can reduce inflammation and others that promote it.

There is still a lot to learn about just how diet and inflammation interact, and research, as of yet, is not at that point where a specific foods or groups of foods can be singled out as being beneficial for people with arthritis. We are beginning to get a clearer picture of how eating the right way can reduce inflammation.

So why are we so concerned about inflammation?

Inflammation is the body's natural defense to infections and injuries. When something goes wrong the body's immune system goes to work to inflame the area, which serves to get rid of the invader or to heal the wound. Inflammation can cause pain, swelling, redness, and warmth, but this goes away as soon as the problem is solved. This is good inflammation.

Then we have chronic inflammation, the type that's familiar to people with rheumatoid arthritis (RA), lupus, psoriatic arthritis, and other types of "inflammatory" arthritis. Chronic inflammation is the type that will not go away.

All the types of arthritis that are mentioned above are a disorder of the immune system creates inflammation and then doesn't know when to shut off. Inflammatory arthritis, chronic inflammation can have serious consequences, permanent disability and tissue damage can be one if it isn't treated properly. Inflammation has been linked to a full host of other medical conditions.

Inflammation has been found to contribute to atherosclerosis, which is when fat builds up on the lining of arteries, raising the risk of heart attacks. Also, high levels of inflammation proteins have been found in the blood of people with heart disease. Inflammation has also been linked to obesity, diabetes, asthma, depression, and even Alzheimer disease and cancer.

Scientists think that a constant level of inflammation in the body, even if the level is low, can have a number of negative effects. Research shows that diet can reduce inflammation; in theory an inflammation-lowering diet should have an effect on a wide range of health conditions.

Researchers have looked for clues in the eating habits of our early ancestors to discover which foods might benefit us the most. They believe those habits are more in tune to our eating habits with how the body processes and uses what we eat and drink.

Our ancestor's diet consisted of wild lean meats (venison or boar) and wild plants (green leafy vegetables, fruits, nuts, and berries). There were no cereal grains until the agriculture revolution (about 10,000 years ago).

There was very little dairy, and there were no processed or refined foods. Our diets are usually are high in meat, saturated (or bad) fats, and processed foods, and there is very little exercise. Nearly everything we eat is available close by or as far away as our computer and the click of a mouse.

Our diet and lifestyles are way out of whack with how our bodies are made from the inside out. While our genetic make-up has changed very little from our early beginnings, our diet and lifestyles have changed a great deal and the changes have gotten worse over the last 50 to 100 years.

Our genes haven't had a chance to adapt. We aren't giving our bodies the right kind of fuel, it's as though we think of our bodies as engines in a jet plane when instead they are like the engine in the very first planes.

There are some foods that we are putting into our bodies, especially because we are eating way too much of them, that are affecting our health in a bad way.

There are two nutrients in our diets that have attracted attention, are omega-3 fatty acids and omega-6 fatty acids have been part of our diets for thousands of years.

They are components in just about all of our many cells and are important for normal growth and development.

Both of these acids play a role in inflammation. In several studies it was found that certain sources of omega 3's in particular, help to reduce the inflammation process and that omega 6's will raise it.

Now this is the problem, the average American eats on average about 15 times more omega 6's than omega 3's.

While our very early ancestor's ate omega 6's and omega 3's in equal ratio, and it is believed that this is what helped to balance their ability to turn inflammation on and off. The imbalance of omega 3's and omega 6's in our diets is believed to contribute to the excess of inflammation in our bodies.

So why is it that we eat so many omega 6's now? Vegetable oils such as corn oil, safflower oil, sunflower oil, cottonseed oil, soybean oil, and the products made from them, such as margarine, are loaded with omega 6's. Even many of the processed snack foods that are so readily available today are full of these oils.

Based on the best information of the time, was to use vegetable oils like those mentioned above instead of foods with saturated fats such as butter and lard. It looks like the consequences of that advice may have contributed to the increased consumption of omega 6's and therefore causing an imbalance of omega 3's and omega 6's.

You can find omega 6's in other common foods such as meats and egg yolks. The omega 6 found in meat is the fatty acids that come from grain-fed animals such as cows, lambs, pigs and chickens.

Most of the meat sold in America is grain fed unlike their grass-fed cousins who contain less of those fatty acids. Wild game such as venison and boar are lower in omega 6's and fat and higher in omega 3's than the meat that comes from the supermarkets where we shop.

You can get omega 3s in both animal and plant food. Our bodies can convert omega 3s from animal sources into anti-inflammatory compounds more easily than the omega 3s from plant sources. Plant foods contain hundreds of other healthful compounds many of which that are anti-inflammatory, so don't discount them all together.

There are many foods that are high in omega 3s and that include fatty fish, especially fish from cold waters. Of course everyone knows about salmon but did you know that you can also find omega 3s in mackerel, anchovies, sardines, herring, striped bass, and bluefish.

It's also widely known that wild fish are better sources of omega 3s than the farm raised ones. You can also buy eggs that have been enriched with omega 3 oils. There are several excellent sources of omega 3s in plants that are leafy greens (like kale, Swiss chard, and spinach) as well as flaxseed, wheat germ, walnuts, and their oils.

You can also get omega 3s in supplements (often as fish oil); this source has been shown to be beneficial in some instances. You should take with your doctor before you take a fish oil supplement because it can interact with some medications and under certain circumstances can increase the risk of bleeding.

I take a prescribed omega 3 supplement because my doctor had told me that the ones you get in the supermarket or health food store are not pure, they have other additives that do absolutely nothing to help.

There are other fats that are contributors to clogged arteries, the "bad" or saturated fats found in meats and high-fat dairy foods, these are called pro-inflammatory.

There are also the Trans fats that are relatively new to the cause of heart disease. These Trans fats can be found in processed convenience and snack foods and can be spotted by reading the labels.

They can be identified as partially hydrogenated oils, often soybean oil or cottonseed oil. But, they can also occur naturally in small amounts in animal foods. The thought is that they contribute to the pro-inflammatory activities in our bodies and the amounts we eat today are staggering.

Antioxidants are substances that prevent inflammation causing "free radicals" from over taking our bodies. Plant foods such as fruits, vegetables (including beans), nuts, and seeds carry high amounts of antioxidants. Extra-virgin olive oil and walnut oil are very good sources of antioxidants, also.

These foods have long been considered the basics for good health, and can be found in fruits and vegetables with colorful and vibrant pigments.

The more colorful the plant, the better they are for you, from green vegetables, especially leafy ones, to low-starch vegetables, such as broccoli and cauliflower, to berries, tomatoes, and brightly colored orange and yellow fruits and vegetables.

We don't have to revert back completely to the caveman to eat the anti-inflammatory way to benefit from the anti-inflammatory diet. Just eating a healthful diet that is recommended today is right on track.

Our chief strategy should be to balance the amount of modern day foods with the foods of long ago, which were rich in the inflammation reducing foods.

Really, all we have to do is replace foods rich in omega 6 with foods rich in omega 3, cutting down on how much meat and poultry we eat while eating oily fish a couple of times a week and adding more varieties of colorful fruits and vegetables, and while whole grains were not a part of our early ancestor's diet, it should be included in ours.

Be sure that it is whole grains and not refined grains because they contain many beneficial nutrients and inflammation-tempering compounds. Researchers have found that eating a lot of foods high in sugar and white flour may promote inflammation, although there is more studying that needs to be done on the subject.

The amounts of knowledge we have on how the body works and how our ancestor's ate is helping to confirm the old adage: "You are what you eat." But, there is still more we need to learn before we can prescribe any one anti-inflammatory diet.

Our genetic makeup and the severity of our health condition will determine the benefits we get from an anti-inflammatory diet and unfortunately there is doubt that there will be one diet that fits us all.

Also, what we eat or don't eat is just a small part of the whole story. We are not as physically active as our ancestors and physical activity has its own anti-inflammatory effects. Our ancestors were also much leaner than we are and body fat is active tissue that can make inflammatory producing compounds.

Anti-inflammatory eating is a way of selecting foods that are more in tune with what the body actually needs. We can achieve a more balanced diet by going back to our roots.

Chapter 4

Biggest Struggles Of An Anti-Inflammatory Diet

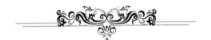

Everyone wants to feel better and live in better health. One of the easiest ways to achieve that is by switching from a traditional western diet to an anti-inflammatory diet. Making the change is easy, but much like a diet plan, sticking with the food changes and watching what you eat can be difficult.

Fast food is a huge hindrance to the anti-inflammatory diet. Foods that are high in fat tend to increase inflammatory substances in the body for three to four hours after the meal.

If the same number of calories eaten in one fast food sitting were eaten as fresh fruits, vegetables and lean meats, this effect would not occur. Free radicals, cell killers that compound inflammation problems, can also be increased by 175% after eating fast food.

The Alternative - The best alternative to fast food is a replacement, anti-inflammatory diet. Take the Big Mac from McDonald's into consideration. This sandwich can be made from lean ground turkey and a whole grain bun.

The "special" sauce can be mixed up with lower carbohydrate ketchup, olive oil mayonnaise and sugar free relish. The result is a tasty alternative with a significantly lower fat count.

Red Meat, Milk and Your Inflammation

Science has long fought to connect red meat with certain forms of cancer. Little did they know the research would lead to a link between this common dinner protein and inflammation. Researchers believe the body reacts to certain chemical aspects of red meat and milk in a protective manner.

If the body believes these are foreign substances, the immune system will kick in and inflammation occurs. Imagine eating red meat once a day and drinking two or three glasses of milk. The body would live in a state of constant or chronic inflammation which could cause health problems over time.

The Alternative - Lean poultry, beef and fish are all part of a healthy diet. Beef is a great source of iron, so eliminating it is not a necessity. But, choosing the leanest of cuts is essential to good health. The best meats are lean proteins and beans.

Trans Fats and Your Inflammation

A hidden source of body inflammation is the trans fatty acid. While many people know a bit about this type of fat, few understand the effects on the body. Fast food, baked goods, prepackaged meals and margarine are often good sources of trans fat.

After entering the body, these fats can increase the risk of coronary artery disease, insulin resistance, diabetes and heart failure. Increased risk of stroke due to abnormally high lipid levels is also common.

While many foods will claim to be trans-fat free, that is not the entire truth. According to labeling guidelines, these foods can contain up to 0.5 grams of trans fats per serving and still mark the product as "trans fat free". These small amounts will add up over time if the diet is rich in processed foods, margarine and baked goods.

Natural fats like whole butter and olive oil have no trans fats. Choosing these in place of hydrogenated oils and margarine is a good first step.

When it comes to foods cooked in trans-fat, there is no choice but to eliminate these from the diet all together. Many people choose to adopt an anti-inflammatory diet by baking their own snacks and cooking "fast food" style meals at home.

Chapter 5

Anti-Inflammatory Foods To Add To Your Diet

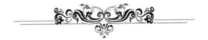

Inflammation is the first sign when something harmful or irritating is affecting parts of our body. Every one's body has an immune system and inflammation is part of that.

Inflammation is also a localized physical condition that results as a reaction to an injury or infection, causing parts of the body to become swollen, reddened, painful and hot. Internal inflammation can happen due to eating of processed foods, fats and sugars.

High levels of inflammation can cause a number of health complications such as arthritis, joint pain, damage to blood vessels among others.

To combat this, it is important you eat foods that are anti-inflammatory. Such foods are readily available to add to your diet to curb inflammation. Here are some of the foods and suggestions to help and keep harmful inflammation at bay:

Whole Grains

When it comes to whole grains it is better you consume your grains as whole grains and not refined or pasta. Research has shown that whole grains contain a high amount of fibre which reduces the inflammatory marker in blood known as C-reactive protein.

Dark Leafy Greens

Dark leafy vegetables such as spinach and kale have high concentrations of vitamin E and minerals such as calcium and iron. Studies show that vitamin E helps in protecting your body from inflammatory molecules known as cytokines. Additionally, dark leafy greens have a high amount of disease fighting phytochemicals.

Fatty Fish

Oily fish such as salmon and tuna are foods that are anti-inflammatory as they contain high amounts of omega 3 fatty acids. The fatty acids are known to help joint inflammation, so make sure you get plenty of omega 3. Another important fact about omega 3 is you must get it in your food because the body cannot make it within its system.

Soy

Soybeans contain isoflavones compounds which help the negative effects of inflammation on joints. However, it is good you avoid heavily processed soy products as they may contain additives and preservatives. Instead, include soy milk and soy beans into your regular diet.

Nuts

Nuts such as almonds and walnuts are rich in vitamin E, calcium and fibre. All nuts are full of antioxidants which can help the body in repairing the damages caused by inflammation.

Berries

Berries are low in fat and calories but rich in antioxidants. Their anti-inflammatory anthocyanins compound in them has many good qualities. This helps to prevent you from developing arthritis.

Green Tea

Green tea as well has anti-inflammatory flavonoids; this reduces the onset of inflammation and minimizes the risk of certain cancers. It shouldn't be underestimated for many other health benefits. It can reactivate skin cells making skin appear brighter. Drink it regularly and use some honey as a sweetener instead of sugar.

Low Fat Dairy

Low fat dairy such as yogurt contains probiotics which can prevent inflammation. Additionally, dairy foods that are anti-inflammatory such as skim milk with high calcium and vitamin D are important for everyone since apart from having anti-inflammatory properties, they strengthen your bones also.

Ginger and Garlic

Ginger and garlic are foods that are anti-inflammatory. Both are known to lower body inflammation, control blood sugar levels and help your body in fighting certain infections. Selenium and sulphur in garlic is an essential compound for a healthy immune system. It is also one of the top anti-aging foods you can eat.

Turmeric and Sweet Potato

Turmeric has natural anti-inflammatory compounds called curcumin which is known to turn off NF-kappa B protein that triggers the process of inflammation. On the other hand, sweet potato is a good source of fibre, vitamin B 6, vitamin C, complex carbohydrates and better carotene.

Wine

It's common knowledge that drinking wine in moderation is a good cardiac-protective activity. A lesser known quality of grape-based or red wine is that it is composed of high concentration of anti-inflammatory properties. To get the same effects, you can also consume fresh grapes since the skin contains the same features.

Olive Oil

Omega-3 is not the only source of fatty acids. It can be found in abundance in olive oil. the best way to utilize this is to cook your vegetables in olive oil. Studies have indicated that compared to raw veggies, those that have been cooked in olive oil produced more anti-inflammatory properties.

All of these anti-inflammatory foods have been touted by experts as being the most comprehensive and effective diet available. While there are other diet plans which offer similar results, depending upon your own personal circumstances, any diet rich in protein, oils and fiber is beneficial.

CHAPTER 6

How The Anti-Inflammatory Diet Can Protect You From Disease

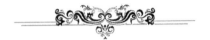

Inflammation is a good thing. It is the natural way your body responds to threats such as infections or wounds. We have all seen inflammation at work when we have pain and redness at an injury. We say it looks inflamed, and it literally is, because injury activates the inflammatory response.

When inflammation lasts for long periods of time, we call it chronic, and it can cause problems. Some common causes of chronic inflammation include allergies, autoimmune disease, periodontal disease, arthritis and other diseases that activate the immune system over time. Even obesity is inflammatory, because fat cells give off chemicals called cytokines that trigger inflammation.

Chronic inflammation causes damage to the endothelial lining of arteries, which can lead to atherosclerosis and heart disease. There is also evidence that it contributes to type 2 diabetes, Alzheimer's disease and a growing number of other chronic diseases that are common in modern, western societies.

The symptoms of inflammation vary with what is causing it. You may even have no symptoms at all, as in the case of obesity. Here are some examples of specific disease related symptoms:

• Arthritis, rheumatoid arthritis (joint pain, stiffness, swelling)

• Crohn's disease or ulcerative colitis (abdominal pain and cramping, fever, diarrhea)

• Psoriasis or eczema (redness)

• Allergies (respiratory symptoms, hives)

More subtle, early indicators of problems could include headaches, muscles aches, fatigue, muscle stiffness, nausea, vomiting, diarrhea or constipation, gas, abdominal discomfort and even emotional problems including depression.

These could be related to food sensitivities and intolerances. The most common food intolerances include dairy (lactose), wheat (gluten), yeast, soy, corn, eggs and even some artificial sweeteners.

You can find out if you have inflammation by having your C- reactive protein levels tested. The high sensitivity C-reactive protein, is the preferred indicator of chronic, low-grade inflammation.

If your C-reactive protein levels are high, you will first want to talk to your doctor to find out if there is an underlying infection, allergy, autoimmune disorder or other contributing disease. If not, your excess weight could be the cause and weight loss is your best line of defense. If you are a smoker, that could also be contributing to the problem.

Inflammation can also be influenced by the foods you eat. Research has shown that certain foods trigger inflammation and others suppress it.

Some of the foods that are pro-inflammatory include:

Animal fats (corn-fed beef, dark meat and skin of poultry, pork, duck

Hydrogenated fats (trans fat)

Fried foods (fried in saturated,hydrogenated or polyunsaturated fats)

Sweets (sugar, candy, cookies, cakes, ice cream, donuts, sweet drinks)

Refined grains (white bread, pasta, white rice)

Processed foods (chips, crackers, fries, cold cuts, hot dogs, canned meats)

Dairy products (especially full fat milk, cheese, sour cream, cream cheese, cream)

Some people may also need to avoid the nightshades (potatoes, tomatoes, eggplant, peppers)

Here are some of the best anti-inflammatory foods:

Fatty fish such as salmon, sardines, herring, trout and tuna (with omega 3 fatty acids)

Grass fed beef also contain some omega 3 fats (unlike corn-fed beef, mostly saturated fats)

Nuts and seeds (walnuts, flaxseed, almonds)

Monounsaturated fats (olive oil, canola oil, avocados), by replacing polyunsaturated fats

Turmeric (part of most curry dishes)

Ginger, used in Asian cuisine (also helps control nausea)

Whole grains (except wheat, barley and rye if you are gluten intolerant)

Foods that have high antioxidant levels also tend to reduce inflammation, possibly by reducing the damage that stimulates inflammation. Antioxidants are prolific in brightly and darkly colored fruits and vegetables.

Some of the best sources of antioxidants include:

Berries: blueberries, raspberries, blackberries, cranberries, strawberries, cherries,

Beans: Red beans, kidney beans, pinto and black beans

Herbs: oregano, basil, sage, marjoram, thyme, dill, garlic, dry mustard

Spices: cinnamon, cloves, cumin, turmeric, ginger

Nuts: pecans, walnuts, pistachios

Green tea is rich in both antioxidants and anti-inflammatory compounds

Coffee, cocoa (or dark chocolate) and red wine (but caffeine and alcohol are inflammatory)

Exotic fruits: acai, gogi, pomegranate, papaya, pineapple

Eating more of these anti-inflammatory and high antioxidant foods can help calm chronic inflammation and by doing so, reduce your risk for chronic diseases. Find ways to make these foods a part of your everyday diet and you will not only be protecting your body from disease, but you may find that some of your aches and pains improve.

Chapter 7

Who Should Eat The Anti-Inflammatory Diet?

Most chronic diseases are a result of a lifestyle of affluence that affords us the luxury of being able to eat the wrong foods in the wrong amounts at the wrong times. These food choices set in play a host of processes in your body that produce inflammation from a multitude of sources.

In addition, many of us are genetically programmed to produce excessive inflammation when exposed to common irritant sources such as smoke, chemicals and poor dietary choices. Some of us produce so much inflammation that we have autoimmune disorders such as lupus, multiple sclerosis, rheumatoid arthritis, psoriasis and colitis.

How exactly do poor food choices produce inflammation?

Packaged and highly processed foods as well as fast foods are some of the worst culprits. They are also some of the food choices most widely available. Designed for convenience, these foods are loaded with trans-fat to extend their shelf life as well as change their taste and texture.

A trans-fat is created from a natural, saturated fat - another less than healthy fat. That saturated fat is "transformed" into a trans-fat via a process called trans-hydrogenation.

This transformed fat is chemically different enough from a natural fat that, when incorporated into your body tissues, it creates a cascade of chemicals called cytokines. Cytokines are molecules responsible for producing inflammation throughout your body.

Foods that are loaded with refined sugars are also inflammatory. Cakes, cookies and doughnuts are examples of foods that are rapidly digested by your body, releasing large amounts of glucose. This glucose is rapidly absorbed by your body, causing a high blood glucose level. Your body in turn releases a surge of insulin to help normalize your blood glucose levels.

This surge of insulin combined with high blood glucose levels causes your body to release cytokines, inflammatory molecules, as well. Each surge of glucose actually signals your body to store fat. Guess what? Fat tissue becomes physiologically active and begins to release these same inflammatory molecules, cytokines, as well.

Refined grains - grains stripped of fiber and vital nutrients- also create inflammation. A whole grain is a molecule composed of large amounts of glucose linked together and encapsulated with a fiber coating. This fiber coating makes the digestion and release of glucose a slow and steady process.

When the outer fiber coating is stripped away to create a smooth and creamy texture, glucose molecules are readily available for rapid digestion and absorption into your body. This rapid surge of glucose into your system again is the trigger for the inflammatory cascade.

Certain grains have the ability to produce inflammation in certain individuals. Wheat, oats, barley and rye are all grains that contain significant amounts of a protein substance called gluten. Gluten makes foods, like bread, crunchy on the outside and soft on the inside.

Yet this same gluten is very inflammatory in individuals genetically challenged in digesting gluten. Symptoms can be as severe as pain, bloating, diarrhea and malnutrition or as mild as nausea or lack of energy. Eliminating these specific grains from your diet is often the key to controlling this type of inflammation.

Inflammation affects every person in the world at some point in their life. In western cultures, like the United States, a huge portion of the population is affected by inflammation every day.

Being overweight or obese is the most common inflammatory condition. It is this inflammatory response that could be the cause of some weight related conditions like diabetes.

When fat cells grow, they take up the free space around the organs. Blood flow can be constricted and the body often feels as though it needs to fight to function normally.

When the body feels threatened, inflammation occurs as a natural, healing response. Unfortunately, unlike the small cut that will heal in a few, short days. Obesity takes time to correct and the longer the body lives inflamed, the greater the risk of long term effects.

In the case of obesity, changing the diet by reducing calories will reduce body weight and thus reduce the inflammation in the body. This is the simplest benefit of an anti-inflammatory diet. However, people who are obese or overweight are not the only people who can benefit from an anti-inflammatory diet.

There are many illnesses and conditions caused by inflammation. These include asthma, arthritis, inflammatory bowel syndrome, pelvic inflammatory disease, endometriosis, diabetes, COPD, Psoriasis, Colitis, and Lupus - just to name a few. All-in-all, there are nearly 40 autoimmune conditions currently accepted by the medical community that are affected by inflammation.

The first step is to make dietary changes to reduce food based inflammation. Processed foods, fast foods and prepackaged foods can cause increased inflammation in the body.

Replacing these foods with lean meats, whole grains and healthy fats will make a tremendous different in how the body reacts to inflammation. In addition, if weight is a problem, reducing weight while changing to an anti-inflammatory diet can increase the benefits exponentially.

Changing to an anti-inflammatory diet does not have to be in reaction to a disease or illness. Prevention is the best choice and the anti-inflammatory diet can reduce the risk of contracting many of the listed illnesses.

When the body feels as though it needs to fight for survival, inflammation occurs, so offering healthy foods that have an inflammatory effect is a great choice for all people including those who are young, healthy and feel they do not need an anti-inflammatory diet.

Chapter 8

Foods Hurting Your Anti-Inflammatory Diet

You have chosen to take your life and your health back and eat an anti-inflammatory diet. Many people are making the same choice to fight the effects of obesity, diabetes, arthritis and other inflammatory conditions. As is the case with any dietary change, after a time, the control once assumed over the foods eaten can grown lax.

Often, the same foods will creep back into the diet and reduce the efficacy of the anti-inflammatory diet. These are packaged foods, oil blends and margarine. Reducing protein and water intake are the remaining common factors.

Packaged foods are just plain bad for the body. Often these foods contain enough sodium and dietary fat for an entire day. While it may seem harmless to pop a meal in the microwave two or three times a week, the impact can be dramatic.

On average, prepackaged meals have between 700 and 1000 calories each. Just three meals a week can contribute an additional 3000 calories to the diet, not to mention the increases in fat and sodium. High fat meals cause inflammation in the body for hours after consumption and can lead to weight gain which is causes more inflammation.

Oil blends are easier on the budget than pure olive oil. These blends, however, can include oils that contain trans fats. These fats are unhealthy and should not be consumed at ALL in the diet. Saving a bit of money on the front side may be counteracting your good anti-inflammatory diet choices on the back side.

Margarine is cheaper and contains fewer calories than butter. Some people even believe that eating pure butter can cause an increase in cholesterol levels which may lead to stroke. This is NOT the case.

People who choose to eat very low carbohydrate diets, which often include high butter intakes, measure lower cholesterol numbers than their margarine or low fat eating peers.

Protein is expensive and lean protein can break the budget. When money is tight, buying that fatty burger to replace the 93/7 lean beef that was part of your anti-inflammatory diet may seem like a harmless choice. Fatty red meat is linked to an increased risk of cancer and causes inflammation in the body. Instead, try replacing the burger, all together, will beans.

Water is the fluid of life and drinking water is the best choice for bettering overall health and decreasing inflammation. Many people start off an anti-inflammatory diet by drinking a half gallon of water a day or more.

Over time, lax behavior may lead to increased caffeine intake and reduced water intake. Caffeine is linked to inflammation and can cause the anti-inflammatory diet to work less effectively at reducing inflammation.

The anti-inflammatory diet is not about strictly forbidding all foods that may increase inflammation. Deprivation is the number one reason people scrap new diets and return to old eating habits. Instead of depriving, try healthier alternatives or simply reduce the number of times prepackaged foods, fatty red meats and trans fat based oils are eaten.

Chapter 9

Anti-Inflammatory Diet Plan

Inflammation triggers a response from the immune system. Initially inflammation is beneficial as it is used for protection but a lot of the time inflammation can lead to further inflammation (Chronic) which leads to big health problems.

There are certain foods contained in many people's diet today which lead to an increase in inflammation. You can probably guess what kinds of foods these are (fake foods, fried foods, processed foods, refined carbs, coffee, alcohol).

The anti-inflammatory diet contains many foods, which I have recommended for other purposes which help to stop and reduce inflammation. It is a very natural way of improving your health and recovering from illness or injury.

Without inflammation to worry about you will be a lot healthier and less at risk of picking up some very harmful illnesses in the long run.

Healthy fats make up a large proportion of the anti-inflammation diet. Foods high in Omega-3 fatty acids have been proven to be anti-inflammatory so I recommend eating as many of these foods to help fight inflammation.

Fish is a great source so stock up on sardines, salmon, herring and anchovies. Other good sources include extra virgin olive oil, coconut oil, avocado oil and walnuts.

Antioxidant Rich Fruit and Vegetables

Fruit and vegetables are packed full of antioxidants and vitamins, some of these vitamins are proven to be anti-inflammatory. Some of the best sources of vegetables include onions, spinach, sweet potato, peppers, garlic, broccoli and other green leafy vegetables.

Good fruits and berries to look out for are blueberries, papaya, pineapple and strawberries. They are packed with high antioxidant content which is great on such a diet.

High Quality Protein

Which proteins you eat are very important. There is a big difference between cheap value meats and grass fed organic meats. The cheap value meats will most likely be packed with hormones and pesticides, which lead to inflammation, whereas grass fed organic meat will help to fight inflammation.

Pick your meat wisely and go for the omega-3 packed grass fed versions as often as you can. Use this rule when it comes to eggs as well. Steak, fish, eggs and poultry and beans (legumes).

These three types of foods form the cornerstone of the anti-inflammation diet.

Also herbs and spices including ginger, curcumin, turmeric, oregano and rosemary contain important substances which reduce inflammation and help to limit dangerous free radical production.

Food to Avoid at All Costs on an Anti-Inflammation Diet

I have just mentioned the foods that can lead to a reduction of inflammation which will keep you healthy. These foods I'm about to mention are the foods which cause inflammation and you should really avoid these.

So if you regularly eat any of the above foods just mentioned then you need to start to cut them out. Eating these types of foods on an anti-inflammation diet completely defeats the purpose of what you are trying to do and will ruin your results.

Even if you don't suffer from inflammation but want to change your eating habits then following this type of diet will still be good for you. It will increase your health greatly and will help with fat loss.

The next steps would be to begin to introduce anti inflammation foods into your diet. Begin with adding the healthy omega 3 fats. Start to use extra virgin olive oil with your vegetables, coconut oil with your cooking, start snacking with nuts instead of chocolate bars and crisps and start to eat more fresh fish. Supplementing with a high quality fish oil supplement is also very important.

Chapter 10

Steps To Start Eating Healthier Today

There are many ways to stop the effect your diet has on inflammation. The easiest is adopting an anti-inflammation diet. Here are the three beginning steps to starting the diet off right.

Fruits, Vegetables and Seafood are good.

Vegetables that offer a deep color are often better for your health. These deep colors often mean higher fiber content and better anti-inflammatory effects on the body. Herbs are also fantastic additions to an anti-inflammation diet. Here is a list of foods and herbs that will best help you to gain control over your inflammation.

- • Turmeric

- • Oregano
- • Garlic
- • Green Tea
- • Blueberries
- • Ginger
- • Wild Seafood
- • Spinach
- • Collard Greens
- • Kale

When choosing seafood, the smaller the fish the better. Mercury is present in all fish and this is a compounding element. Eating the smaller fish like sardines, means eating from the lower end of the food chain with less mercury.

The idea is to boost healthy foods and eliminate unhealthy foods so for every good food you choose as part of your anti-inflammation diet, try taking out a processed food or fatty meat.

Increase Essential Fatty Acids (EFAs)

There is talk all over the Internet and in print about the power of EFAs. These fatty acids are present in nearly every food we eat, but the ratio of the different fatty acids is important as well as general consumption. Most people consume far more Omega 6s than Omega 3s and that can reduce the healthiness of even the best anti-inflammation diet.

Foods rich in Omega 3s include fish oil, olive oil, avocado, walnuts and grapeseed oil. An Omega 3 supplement can also be taken to boost this EFA in the diet. While flaxseed oil is the best source of Omega 3s, a fish oil supplement can also be chosen. It is important to make sure the fish oil is mercury free and tested for heavy metals.

Nuts and seeds are also perfect sources of EFAs. There is nothing hard about adding a handful of nuts or seeds to a salad or as a snack every day. For people with nut allergies, soy provides a healthy alternative. Soy is also a good source of lean protein which also has an anti-inflammation effect.

You may also hear about Omega 9 fatty acids. These are naturally occurring in the body, but that does not mean the amounts of this EFA when compared to Omega 3 and Omega 6 should not be taken into consideration. The effect of EFAs is heavily dependent on balance.

So far, stepping into an anti-inflammation diet has been really easy. During the elimination phase, however, some people have trouble giving up the foods they have grown to love the most. When listing the foods that need to be eliminated for their inflammatory effect on the body in order of importance, the list would include:

- • Trans Fats
- • Sugar
- • Refined Carbohydrates
- • Potential Food Allergens

Trans fats are present in hydrogenated oils like margarine. Despite many labels ready "0 trans fats"; they are still in those products in small amounts. Sugar is just not good for the body.

Replacing processed sugar with natural cane may be a healthier alternative. Refined carbohydrates include processed flour which is used in nearly every loaf of bread and baked goods sold in a package. Try baking for yourself with whole grain flour instead.

Food allergens often include gluten, soy, eggs, dairy and nuts. These foods will increase inflammation in the body immediately if there is a food allergy.

Medical food allergy testing can provide a specific list of food that will cause a reaction in the body. If you want to find out which foods you are allergic to on your own, keep a journal and eliminate the foods one by one for a few days.

Then, eat the food in question to see if there is a change or reaction. Mild food allergies often affect gastrointestinal systems with constipation or diarrhea. Rashes and hives, both inflammatory responses, may also appear.

Chapter 11

How To Cure Sciatica With An Anti-Inflammatory Diet

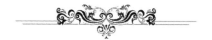

Increased consumption of processed foods has led directly to an increase in pain and discomfort related to inflammation in the body, including sciatica. Sciatica occurs when inflammation puts pressure on the sciatic nerve, causing pain in the lower back and down one or both legs. Foods rich non-inflammatory qualities are one answer for how to cure sciatica at home.

Inflammation is the body's natural reaction to injury or infection. It can be beneficial when the systems of the body are working to repair themselves. However, modern diets have led to an abundance of inflammation without a purpose, which poses a variety of problems.

Many people use NSAIDs, or anti-inflammatory medications such as ibuprofen, to relieve pain from inflammation. However, most do not consider the risks of NSAID overuse.

The most common issue that arises from using anti-inflammatory drugs is gastrointestinal pain. In serious cases, long-term NSAID users experience fatal ulcers and other life-threatening ailments. An anti-inflammatory diet is an alternative to medication.

How to Cure Sciatica at Home with an Anti-inflammatory Diet:

1. Eat anti-inflammatory foods. Kelp, Wild Alaskan Salmon, Turmeric, Shitake Mushrooms, Papaya, Blueberries, Broccoli, and Sweet Potatoes are some popular anti-inflammatory foods. Not only will these foods help reduce swelling, thereby, decreasing pain, they will also provide balanced nutrition and taste great.

2. Drink anti-inflammatory drinks. Drinking plenty of water and green tea will reduce swelling, redness, and

discomfort associated with inflammation. Adults should drink 8 glasses of water per day.

Water will have the added benefits of reducing appetite and clearing skin. In addition to reducing inflammation, green tea has also been shown to decrease the risks of cancer and heart disease.

3. Cook with Extra Virgin Olive Oil. EVOO is the Mediterranean secret to good health. The abundant supply of polyphenols is vital in reducing inflammation in the heart and blood vessels. The monounsaturated fats in olive oil are used by the body as anti-inflammatory agents, decreasing asthma and rheumatoid arthritis.

4. Supplement fish oils. If you are not eating 2 portions of oily fish per week, use fish oil supplements to decrease inflammation. You are looking for 2-3 grams a day of EPA and DHA. Ginger and turmeric supplements are also very beneficial to your health.

If you have been experiencing chronic pain, try an anti-inflammatory diet before use of risky medications or invasive surgeries. If you have been looking for an answer for how to cure sciatica at home, start with sensible food choices.

Additionally, you should try increasing the amount of exercise you are doing regularly. Walking and stretching are ideal ways to relieve pain.

Chapter 12

The Anti-Inflammatory Diet For Arthritis Relief

Food and arthritis have a connection to each other and that is why changing your diet is one of the first pieces of advice an expert can give a person with inflammation in his or her joints. There are foods that can reduce inflammation and there are those that might worsen the inflammation.

A person with arthritis should follow the anti-inflammatory diet if he or she wants to get treated. To start an anti-inflammatory diet, one should know which foods he or she going to eliminate in one's diet and which foods will be added.

What are the foods that you should avoid and eliminate in your diet? When it comes to arthritis, it is always advised that the person affected should eliminate artificial foods like junk foods, those foods that have been processed and foods with added artificial flavorings and colorings.

A person with arthritis should also avoid meats that have high levels of fats and foods that are high in sugar. The reasons why these kinds of foods should be avoided by people with arthritis is that the saturated fats and trans fats found in these kinds of foods can worsen one's condition.

He or she should also avoid potatoes, eggplants and tomatoes because these are part of the nightshade family of plant that contains solanine that can provoke the pain.

Cutting these kinds of vegetables in people with arthritis have not been proven yet to be effective, but those who followed this kind of diet often show improvements with their condition and find relief from pain.

What are the foods to be added in your diet if you have arthritis? If you already know which kinds of foods you should eliminate in your anti-inflammatory diet, you should now know foods to add to your diet:

1. Healthy fats and Oils: Fish oils are high in Omega-3 fatty acids that are essential to our health. This will help reduce the inflammation and prevent it from coming back. You will also get these fats in some seeds like flaxseed, pumpkin seeds, and sunflower seeds and also in Brazil nuts, almonds, cashew nuts and many more.

2. Fruits and Vegetables: You should be eating more fruits and vegetables if you have arthritis because these have a lot of mineral, vitamins, antioxidants and photochemical that are beneficial for your arthritis and also to other conditions.

3. Protein: Eating more proteins like fishes and other seafoods and poultry meats will also help people with arthritis.

4. Drinks: You should need more liquids to keep your joints lubricated. Drink more water, fruit juices, tea, vegetable juice with low sodium and non-fat milk.

Chapter 13

Anti-Inflammatory Diet For Treating Our Nail Fungus

The anti-inflammatory diet can help boost your immune system, which can help fight off fungal infections. Drinking the recommended six to eight glasses of water a day is suggested with this diet, which can help to cleanse your inner system, also helping to fight off infection.

In addition to being helpful in the fight to rid oneself of a fungus infection, there are other health benefits attached to the diet such as help with depression and improved mental state, a stronger immune system, less water retainage and more.

The anti-inflammatory diet usually consists of eating 2,000 to 3,000 calories a day. The amount of calories depends on your size. You should be eating 40 to 50% of carbohydrates, 30 % of fat and include carbohydrates, fat and protein with each meal.

This diet uses a lot of fish and fresh fruits and vegetables while minimizing the consumption of fast food meals. Beans, winter squashes and sweet potatoes are also a big part of this diet. This diet is not typically meant for weight loss, but can be used for health reasons and is said to help with fungal problems.

It may take a little while for the diet to work. Remember, if you've been eating a totally different diet, particularly if it was a poor diet, it will take a while for your system to be completely cleaned out. You might want to make a visit to a nutritionist or to the local health food store to discuss how and when the diet will work.

You can expect any treatment to take six to twelve weeks to work and the change in your diet alone may not be enough. Keep a journal of what you eat and do and any changes you see if you are unsure of the effectiveness of treatment.

Again, this is something to be discussed with your healthcare physician, a dietitian or nutritionist or even your health foot store representative who is well-versed in dietary needs.

At times, a health foot store may have different or more reliable information than the internet or even your physician's office and may be able to give you some supplements, topical creams or organic lacquers which may prove to be extremely effective, especially in conjunction with the anti-inflammatory diet.

Chapter 14

How To Lose Weight And Feel Great With The Anti-Inflammatory Diet

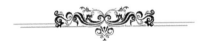

The anti-inflammatory diet can make you feel great. "How," you ask. By cutting out or significantly reducing your consumption of pro-inflammatory foods. When these foods are cut from your diet, inflammation in the body reduces taking stress and strain from the joints and organs.

While following this diet your chance of weight loss also goes up. "How does this happen," by reducing your consumption of grain and wheat products, sodas, and other simple sugars that cause excess weight.

In short summary, the fewer inflammatory foods we eat, the less inflammation we have in the body.

Background Information on Pro-Inflammatory Foods:

Grains, refined sugars, partial-hydrogenated oils, vegetable and seed oils are from modern man. These foods have been around a short time; hence, obesity and disease are on the rise. Humans are genetically adapted to eat fruits, veggies, nuts, lean meats, and fish, foods not related to chronic diseases.

Why Do Grains Inflame?

Grains contain a protein called gluten. Gluten is the main cause of many digestive diseases, such as celiac disease, also contributor to frequent headaches.

They also have a sugar protein called lectins which has been shown to cause inflammation in the digestive system. Grains also contain phytic acid which is known to reduce the body's absorption of calcium, magnesium, iron, and zinc.

Lastly, grains contain high amounts of fatty acid biochemicals called omega-6 fatty acids which do cause inflammation. Fatty acid biochemicals known as omega-

3 fatty acids are anti-inflammatory and found in fresh fish and green vegetables.

What Should I Eat?

Anti-inflammatory foods

All fruits and vegetables (raw or lightly cooked)

Red and sweet potatoes

Anti-inflammatory omega-3 eggs

Raw nuts

Spices such as ginger, turmeric, garlic

Organic butter, coconut oil, extra virgin olive oil

Fresh fish, avoid farm raised

Meat, chicken, eggs from grass-fed animals

Wild game such as deer, elk, etc.

Water, organic green tea, red wine, stout beer

Chapter 15

Anti-Inflammatory Diet To Slow Down Cellular Aging

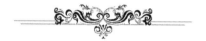

Chemical oxidation of cells is a natural process for the body. However, these have some bad effects to the DNA and to electrons. When the cells undergo energy conversion process, the body produces harmful free radicals.

These free radicals are single electrons that follow a unique path. When they meet paired electrons in your system, they snatch one of the paired electrons. This leads to cellular inflammation and DNA damage.

Cellular inflammation plays a huge role in the accelerated process of skin aging. Wrinkles appear faster and skin tissues become more fragile. Eventually, this leads to the loss of dermis elasticity. Thin skin condition and saggy dermis are just some of the problems you might have to deal with in the future.

One of the best ways to prevent cellular aging is to have an anti-inflammatory diet. Basically, foods rich in antioxidants are consumed. Antioxidants are molecules that fight harmful free radicals. These molecules also prevent the formation of free radicals.

Here are some tips on how to slow down cellular aging:

1. Instead of eating junk foods for your snack, eat dark colored berries instead. Blackberries, blueberries and raspberries contain a hefty amount of antioxidants that can fight cellular aging. In addition to that, they are also rich sources of vitamins and minerals that can help fight the over-all skin aging process.

2. Always have vegetable side dishes for your main meals. Green leafy vegetables are rich sources of antioxidative molecules. They can further avoid cellular aging.

3. Increase your intake of cold water fish like Tuna and Salmon. They are the best sources of omega-3 fatty acids DHA and EPA. According to experts, nothing can prevent cellular inflammation more than omega-3 fatty acids. These fatty acids prevent inflammatory problems of any kind. This can even reduce joint inflammation so you can have better health.

A good diet is fundamental to young looking skin. But in addition to that, you also need to feed your skin with a natural moisturizer that contains beneficial ingredients like CynergyTK, Phytessence Wakame and Nano Lipobelle HEQ10.

CynergyTK is an ingredient found in the wool of sheep. This ingredient is made up of functional keratin, a complex type of protein needed for the production of collagen. Phytessence Wakame is a type of sea kelp that can prevent the sudden loss of hyaluronic acid.

This acid is essential for collagen lubrication. Nano Lipobelle HEQ10 is an antioxidant that can further avoid cellular inflammation. This has smaller molecular properties so it can easily penetrate the skin.

Chapter 16

How To Beat Inflammation Naturally

Most people who experience inflammation have heard all about the medications that are available to cure the pain and swelling that can occur during a flare up.

But how many know that there are some great anti-inflammatory foods that can affect how you feel and reduce the pain associated with inflammation. Following an anti-inflammatory diet will help you beat inflammation naturally.

Inflammation is a swelling that may cause pain, discoloration and even the loss of movement. Usually most people experience severe inflammation when they are the sufferers of arthritis and when they have problems like heart disease and strokes.

Usually your doctor will recommend that you get sleep and exercise in moderation. He may also suggest lowering your weight and taking steroid based drugs or undergoing joint replacement surgery.

The medications do work fairly well in reducing the inflammation but often come with some serious side effects, such as ulcers and kidney problems. This may make you wonder if they are worth taking and whether using them is trading one illness for another.

Just like there are some foods that decrease inflammation, there are some that will increase the likelihood that you will get inflammation. These foods are junk foods, fast foods, sugar, and fatty meats.

Processed foods that contain Trans and saturated fats also increase the risk of inflammation. Other large contributors of saturated fats are dairy products and eggs.

By simply choosing low fat milk, low fat cheese and leaner cuts of meat, you can lower the risks of inflammation, as well as cut down on the chances of chronic disease and obesity. Other foods that increase inflammation include presweetened cereals and soft drinks.

In addition to these, there are foods that are high in sugar and foods that come from the plants labeled as nightshade type. These add to the risk of discomfort associated with inflammation.

Eating whole fruits and vegetables will give you the natural healing factors. However, not all vegetables work that way. Potatoes, eggplant and tomatoes can actually make inflammation worse.

In general, eat an abundance of fresh vegetables and fruits, whole grains, anti-inflammatory fats and nuts while limiting processed foods, meat protein, milk products, refined sugars, artificial colors/flavors/sweeteners and food sensitivities.

Vegetables:

Eat and Enjoy:

Enjoy an abundance of fresh vegetables and fruits in a variety of colors (preferably organic). Fruits and vegetables are full of vitamins, minerals, antioxidants and fiber which give the body the essential building blocks for health.

Examples include beans, squash, lintels, sweet potatoes, cruciferous vegetables, avocados, dark leafy greens... There are so many choices. As for fruits, pineapple and papaya are particularly good because they are high in bromelain, a powerful natural anti-inflammatory. Fruits and vegetables also make great, healthy snacks.

Avoid / Limit:

Avoid produce that is not grown organically. Toxic chemical residues from herbicides and pesticides can remain and when ingested are foreign irritants to the system. Many crops in North America are also genetically engineered and are put on the market without rigorous scientific study to determine safety for human consumption.

Independent research is finally being done to show toxic effects of consuming genetically modified organisms (2). Foreign DNA is randomly inserted into the genome of a crop. Examples include herbicide resistant corn and soy which are resistant to the herbicide Roundup, made by Monsanto. Roughly 90% of all corn and soy sold in North America is genetically modified.

Also be aware of derivatives of genetically modified ingredients (such as corn starch and corn syrup etc.). It has also been suggested that consuming GMOs is a contributing factor to the rise in allergies as our bodies are recognizing these food substances as foreign (3). By choosing items with the "certified organic" label, you avoid both GMOs and toxic herbicides/pesticides.

For some people, vegetables in the nightshade family may pose a concern. Examples of nightshade vegetables include tomatoes, peppers, potatoes and eggplant.

Nightshades contain alkaloids which are thought to exacerbate inflammation and joint damage in certain susceptible individuals with arthritis (though research is conflicting). Thus, for some individuals, limiting or avoiding nightshade vegetables may be beneficial.

Fats:

Eat and Enjoy:

Enjoy healthy, anti-inflammatory fats including olive oil, coconut oil, avocados, nuts, salmon and sardines. In humans, there are two essential fatty acids, alpha-linolenic acid (an omega-3) and linoleic acid (an omega-6). These are "essential" because they are required for good health but the body does not synthesize them. Omega-3 fats are anti-inflammatory.

Omega-6 fats can be pro-inflammatory or anti-inflammatory (as it can be metabolized by two different pathways). Researchers suggest that keeping the ratio of omega-6 to omega-3 between 2:1 and 4:1 is best for health.

The modern diet tends to be high in omega-6 as it is abundantly available in cooking oils. Thus, including rich sources of omega-3 is important (such as fish, flax and walnuts especially).

Avoid / Limit:

Fats to limit or avoid include margarine, butter, shortening, hydrogenated oils, trans fats, saturated fats, and milk fat. Omega-6 fats are very high in corn oil, safflower oil and sunflower oil. Trans fats are linked with inflammatory diseases (4).

Meat:

Eat and Enjoy:

In general, limit animal proteins because they tend to acidify the body and also promote inflammation. When selecting animal protein, enjoy fish, poultry (especially free-range and organically raised), lamb and omega-3 eggs.

Avoid / Limit:

Limit beef, pork, shellfish and factory farmed eggs. In general, grass-fed is superior to grain-fed. Avoid charred foods, smoked foods and cold cuts. Cold cuts contain nitrates and nitrites which promote cancer. Barbequed foods contain polycyclic aromatic hydrocarbons (PAHs) and heterocyclic amines (HCAs) which also promote cancer.

Dairy:

Eat and Enjoy:

Enjoy dairy substitutes in moderation (such as almond milk).

Avoid / Limit:

Avoid or limit dairy products in general. This includes milk, yogurt, cheese and ice cream. As we age, we lose the enzyme that digests dairy, resulting in lactose intolerance and inflammation. The milk protein, casein, is also acidifying which (despite what many people are brought up thinking) robs the bones of calcium.

Grains:

Eat and Enjoy:

Enjoy whole grains as opposed to refined grains. Refined grains are grains in which the germ and bran have been removed. This means there is loss of fiber, minerals and vitamins. In other words, the good stuff is removed in exchange for a longer shelf life. Some good examples of healthy grains include (organic) whole wheat/oats/bulgar/coucous, quinoa and whole oats (like steel-cut oats).

Whole grains are also a rich source of complex carbohydrates. Complex carbohydrates (as opposed to simple sugars) will prevent spikes in your blood sugar level. Sugar promotes inflammation.

Avoid / Limit:

Avoid or limit refined carbohydrates such as white bread, pastries, sweet things and pastas.

Nuts:

Eat and Enjoy:

Enjoy nuts and nut butters such as almonds, walnuts, sesame seeds, pumpkin seeds and flax.

Avoid / Limit:

Avoid any specific nut allergies.

Beverages:

Eat and Enjoy:

Enjoy plenty of pure, filtered water (avoiding chlorine, fluoride and other contaminants which are irritants that promote inflammation). Other great choices are lemon water and herbal teas.

Avoid / Limit:

Avoid sugary sodas, fruit juice (with sugar added) and milk.

Spices:

Eat and Enjoy:

Many spices reduce inflammation. Some great examples are turmeric, oregano, rosemary, ginger, garlic and cinnamon. Bioflavenoids and polyphenols reduce inflammation and fight free radicals. Cayenne pepper is also anti-inflammatory, as it contains capsicum. Capsicum is often used in pain-relief creams.

Sweeteners:

Eat and Enjoy:

Enjoy stevia, molasses, maple syrup or honey as better alternatives for refined sugar.

Avoid / Limit:

Avoid refined sugar, fructose and especially high fructose corn syrup which promote inflammation. Avoid artificial sweeteners.

Other:

Eat and Enjoy:

Enjoy fermented foods such as kimchi, miso soup and sauerkraut. Fermented foods are probiotic and help to rebuild the immune system by supporting healthy microflora in the gut and to reduce inflammation. Fermented foods also tend to be easy to digest and are also factories for B vitamins.

Avoid / Limit:

In general, eliminate processed foods, artificial colors, artificial flavors and preservatives. Also avoid foods that you have a known sensitivity or allergy to as this promotes inflammation.

Low grade sensitivities are easy to miss, so if you're unsure, have a food allergy test. Some of the most common problem foods include wheat (gluten), corn, soy, milk and nuts.

Chapter 17

Anti-Inflammatory Herbs And Natural Sources

The concept of anti-inflammatory herbs is s very interesting one in the world of naturopathy and natural health. The reason why I gravitate towards them is because in the realm of inflammation and anti-inflammatory diets, they're a nice middle ground. Some people call for a total anti-inflammatory diet, eating only foods that promote the quelling of inflammation in the body.

Others are on the Standard American Diet, eating a host of foods that are known to cause inflammation in the body and aggravate many disorders and conditions. Anti-inflammatory herbs are a nice in-between. Foods in general are said to be either pro inflammatory or anti-inflammatory.

As you might have guessed, foods that are pro inflammatory will increase the amount of inflammation occurring in different parts of your body, will increase the pain associated with it, and may also increase your risk of having chronic disease. Foods pro inflammatory are most junk foods, sugars, fast foods, highly processed foods, and meats high in fat.

But that seems a bit excessive. That's why I love the idea of anti-inflammatory herbs. They're a nice middle ground in the world of inflammation, allowing you to stay healthy in that arena without putting too much of a focus on inflammation in general.

Regularly eating some form of natural anti-inflammatory foods is key because it helps reduce the risk of things like arthritis and chronic autoimmune diseases. And due to the fact that herbal concoctions are generally fairly strong, anti-inflammatory herbs are a great addition to meals, as well as in supplements.

Herbs generally have a wide variety of health benefits, and because inflammation is a somewhat complex process in the body, herbs can affect inflammation in different ways. Inflammation, when carried beyond reasonable limits, can become a type of autoimmune condition.

It begins as negative stimuli causes white blood cells to activate in order to protect the area being negatively affected. Inflammation is necessary to the healing process, but chronic inflammation can cause lots of long term problems and is often excessive, like an allergic reaction.

Here are some of the best, most powerful anti-inflammatory herbs:

1. Turmeric. Turmeric is a spice very common to most Indian foods. Though it has many other medicinal benefits, turmeric is a powerful anti-inflammatory herbs. But it takes a bit of time to start working, so if you don't like the taste of turmeric, you might want to think about taking it in capsule form.

2. Ginger. Ginger is also a spice that is used very often in Asian cooking. This spice also has a potent flavor and takes a bit of time in order to take effect within the body.

Ginger is very versatile, being used in a range of both foods and drinks, so filling your diet with it shouldn't be too much of a challenge. You can drink ginger tea, ginger ale, use ginger in baked goods and spice meats with it.

3. Omega 3 Essential Fatty Acids. Though these aren't technically herbs, omega 3 essential fatty acids are something that everyone needs more of in their diets. They're not only anti-inflammatory, they have a range of other medicinal benefits all across the body.

4. Licorice. Licorice is another herb that is very effective in the world of anti-inflammation. This too is a great herb to take because of its diversity. Licorice is nice because it can be added to just about anything, like candy, tea, baked goods, vegetables, meats, and more, making it easy to get a high daily dose.

5. Mangosteen Juice. Mangosteen is a fruit native to Asia that has very powerful anti-inflammatory properties.

Mangosteen juice is becoming more and more popular with persons who are suffering from the pain of arthritis, and mangosteen even has a very nice flavor. Many people substitute it for orange juice in their morning breakfast.

A few others worthy of note are:

- Pineapple juice
- Chamomile
- Black Seed Oil
- White Willow
- Red and Black Pepper
- St John's Wort
- Cilantro
- Cinnamon
- Garlic
- Cloves

Chapter 18

Omega-3 Anti-Inflammatory Supplements

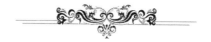

An omega-3 anti-inflammatory supplement is a natural nutritional supplement that has omega-3 fatty acids as its nutrient and benefits source, which is significant because omega-3 has very strong properties from being able to reduce and also inhibit inflammation.

Taking a supplement to manage inflammation is very beneficial because of the importance in keeping excess inflammation from building up in your body and becoming a chronic condition.

If this happens you will largely increase your risks for many different serious health problems, including an increased risk of heart disease and dying from a heart attack.

Additionally, joint problems and arthritis are a common condition, with millions of people suffering from their symptoms, and would very much benefit from an omega-3 anti-inflammatory supplement.

Where Does Omega-3 Come From?

Omega-3 is found in many plants and animals, but there are a few things that are significant to note:

(1) Omega-3 are essential fatty acids, meaning that people need them but they are not made by our bodies, so the must be ingested through diet or supplements.

(2) Omega-3 is not a single fatty acid but a group of fatty acids.

(3) All omega-3 fatty acids do not have the same anti-inflammatory properties.

Keeping these things in mind, the omega-3 fatty acids that have the strongest anti-inflammatory benefits come from omega-3 DHA, with fish oil from cold water fish and green lipped mussels probably being the 2 best sources. On the other hand omega-3 ALA, which is found in plants like flax, does not have inflammation reducing properties.

You especially hear about fish oil omega-3 supplements related to heart health. These are recommended by many heart health professionals, and the American Heart Association strongly recommends for people to increase the amount of fish in their diets - although this would be healthy and a good idea, getting the fish oil from a supplement will give a higher concentration source and further maximize the benefits.

For those with joint problems and arthritis, the green lipped mussel supplement omega-3 is likely more effective.

Like the fish oil, the green lipped mussel will be a very good source for the omega-3 DHA anti-inflammatory, but the mussel supplements will also include omega-3 ETA. This fatty acid is a COX-2 inhibitor, which will help inhibit or keep inflammation from returning to your joints after it is reduced or eliminated.

So, when you start an omega-3 anti-inflammatory supplement, you will want to look at green lipped mussel supplements or fish oil supplements, with part of the decision being related to the specific reason for wanting a supplement to get rid of inflammation - but actually, if you will take both of these together you will receive synergistic benefits, and have the most effective anti-inflammatory alternative.

Chapter 19

Natural Anti Inflammatory Foods For Better Health And Less Pain

Inflammation is recognized by pain, swelling, redness and heat around the affected area. There are different options to treat inflammation. One is medicines, which so far hasn't been most successful because it doesn't really cure the problem.

The other option is the natural way, from where our body originates from; our body been made by nature and gets its natural products from nature.

This means selecting the food that your body needs, because shortfalls of some ingredients most likely caused the illness in the first place. It is also understood our body can react different to foods, because some foods being metabolized different to others.

What that means, as in inflammation some foods can have a positive or a negative result. Here are some of the natural anti-inflammatory foods; if selected correctly they will make that difference in healing.

Natural Anti Inflammatory Foods

Vegetables and fruits: Vegetables and fruits of green and bright colour help the process of inflammatory conditions. Vegetables and fruits are rich in antioxidants such as vitamins, minerals, fibre which the body needs every day to stay healthy.

There are many varieties, per example, squash, sweet potatoes, avocados, beans, lentils, dark green leafy vegetables and cruciferous vegetables. All of these have many antioxidants, phytochemicals and anti-inflammatory properties present.

Important Fats

Also rich in anti-inflammatory foods are olive oil, coconut oil, salmon, sardines, and avocados. All of them contain omega 3 fatty acids which are essential for inflammation and joint health. The acid from omega 3 is an inflammatory agent that changes into prostaglandins which is a hormone like substance.

Omega 3 is not only beneficial for joint pain and inflammation, it is also important for health in general. We only can get omega from our diet, therefore it is important to include some of the healthy oils such olive, coconut, macadamia and krill, which is stronger than fish oil. There are many options of foods available which contain a variety of omega.

Oils you should know about

Olive oil has more health benefits than most people realise. Make sure to use it in your diet as much as possible. Olive oil is high in antioxidants and is containing a substance called oleuropein. Medical science has determined that extra virgin olive oil is one of the healthiest foods we can add to our diet.

This oil is most helpful and effective for arthritis sufferers because it can cool inflammation and ease joint pain. However, for cooking, frying, baking etc. use only coconut or macadamia nut oil.

Other oils when heated become toxic and usually turn into trans fats which can trigger inflammation and joint pain, as well as other health issues. Avoid these oils: Vegetable oils, soy bean, canola, these are the more common ones most people know about because of the names. Yes, they have a healthy sounding name, but they are not healthy.

Spices

Turmeric would be on top of the list in reducing inflammation and joint pain. As well turmeric has a compound curcumin which is known for many health benefits and has the power to cure joint pain. It is best used in its natural powdery form and added to your diet when possible, the more the better.

Other important spices used for reducing inflammation are cinnamon, rosemary, garlic, ginger and oregano. These are high in polyphenols and bioflavonoids which help to reduce inflammation as well as fight off free radicals. Cayenne pepper is also known for its anti-inflammatory property and its capsicum content which is added to some creams for pain relief.

Grain

Whole grains which contain carbohydrates can also help in preventing spikes in the sugar level of the blood, as it is known that sugar promotes inflammation.

However, use only non-refined whole grains, once processing has taken place all the goodness is lost, such as vitamins, minerals and fibre. Among the best grains are oats: Whole oats, whole wheat, quinoa, couscous and Bulgar.

To take a multi supplement is of benefit, it can fill the spot of some foods you otherwise may not get from your diet as needed daily. However, your first priority must always be the diet, only than when taking a supplement you will get best value.

The right type of food and supplementation is crucial to treat arthritis, inflammation and joint pain. Multi vitamins that contain vitamin C, E, zinc, B 6, copper and boron are good to have included in your diet.

It has been found that some nutrients deficiency in patients could be the cause of suffering from arthritis. There is also strong evidence that exercise is just as important as your diet.

Anyone suffering with arthritis pain, the last thing you would think about is exercise. You avoid moving as little as possible because every time you move it creates pain.

In fact, exercise is the alternative to joint pain relief, because it breaks the tendency to favour your joints and to avoid movement. Avoidance of movement and exercise will ultimately make the pain worse and weakens the body.

Chapter 20

Tips For Practicing The Anti-Inflammatory Diet

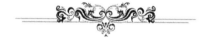

Inflammation and aging go hand in hand as inflammation markers especially the ESR (erythrocyte sedimentation rate) - slowly increase with each decade.

Many age-related diseases have inflammation as their common denominator and this is partially modulated by diet, so here are 10 easy tips to avoid the buildup of damaging inflammation products as much as possible:

Skip the sugar. Diabetes is the classical model of accelerated aging and sugar is made of empty calories anyway. The drive to consume glucose is innate, I know, but choose fresh fruit salads instead. You will get your sugar fix and some nutrients on the side.

The sweet tooth is the part most people find difficult about leading a healthy lifestyle and most traditional sweets are made of eggs, milk, butter and flour which are baked in the oven. That is the perfect recipe for advanced glycation end-products: you have proteins, sugar and high temperatures.

The result is the Maillard reaction. We already 'bake' from within as time passes by, so why add more glycation? You could try raw vegan desserts in exchange. These are made with nuts, seeds and fruits and don't involve any heating or baking, hence they are faster to make as well.

Lately, raw vegan cake shops have started to spring up everywhere. If there is no such place where you live, search online for raw vegan dessert recipes, especially if you have a weakness for sweets. Don't let a day pass without eating a salad and add as many different fresh ingredients to it as possible.

Avoid smoked meat and cheese. Same for grilled meats. In both cases you have the unhappy mix of high temperatures and proteins which easily get denatured. The consumption of these types of products is linked to digestive cancers in populations where they are consumed in high quantity.

There are better ways to prepare animal products, so why risk it? You could try marinated fish or non-smoked fermented cheese. Eat as few animal products as possible - once per week should be enough.

Use the lowest possible temperatures when cooking. If you are baking peppers, you could use a lower temperature and a longer time than if you would bake meat. Of course, you don't want to eat raw meats and get infections. Just use your best judgment when cooking.

Use high moisture levels when cooking. It's much better to boil and broil than to roast or fry ingredients. If you are a fan of crispy food, that would be difficult to implement. On the other hand, there are many fresh vegetables and fruits that are naturally crispy if you feel the need for it - peppers anyone?

You don't need oil to cook. A ceramic pan/pot and a little bit of water will do and food will not stick. Cleaning is a breeze afterwards.

Avoid heating up fats. You can always add cheese, avocado, nuts and seeds in your recipes later on. Don't bake, fry or roast these. Cheese will melt anyway if you place it over steamy fresh potatoes and the end result will be just as delicious.

Water should be your default beverage. Everything else - soups, teas, etc - is a bonus and they will never replace water, even if the human body will work with what is available and it will extract water from them.

People get more dehydrated with age anyway and many substances precipitate if you don't drink enough water, so why speed things up when water is so freely available and cheap? I guess if you are able to read this post, then access to clean water is not an issue. Unfortunately, that's not the case for everybody.

Eat as fresh as possible. If you want to eat meat or seafood, get it fresh and only use frozen ingredients if nothing else is available. Don't cook more food than you eat in one sitting. Heated food is not as fresh or delicious as readily prepared one.

Chapter 21

7 practical recipes throughout the week

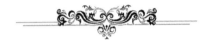

Weekly program

Monday:

Breakfast: Green tea with ginger wholemeal bread and blackberry jam

Snack: 100% blueberry juice

Lunch: Mixed vegetables seasoned with a drizzle of olive oil;

Snack: 50 grams of nuts

Dinner: anchovy pie with beetroot

Tuesday:

Breakfast: Half a cup of whole grains or oats

Snack: A seasonal fruit

Lunch: Whole curry risotto

Snack: White yogurt with live milk enzymes

Dinner: Grilled salmon on a bed of mixed vegetables seasoned with a drizzle of olive oil.

Wednesday:

Breakfast: Infusion of ginger semolina bread and currant jam

Snack: An apple

Lunch: Onion soup, rye bread and fennel bread

Snack: Two squares of dark chocolate

Dinner: Mackerel with lemon and green beans

Thursday:

Breakfast: Green tea or freshly squeezed orange juice

Snack: 6 almonds

Lunch: plenty of vegetables and a spoonful of extra virgin olive oil

Snack: 125 grams of low-fat yogurt with little pieces of fruit

Dinner: Lentil balls and lettuce side dish

Friday:

Breakfast: bread or rusks or biscuits or cereals

Snack: a seasonal fruit

Lunch: cooked or raw vegetables

Snack: fruit ice cream

Dinner: 120 grams of turkey or defatted chicken

Saturday:

Breakfast: Rusks or 1 wholemeal sandwich / rye or whole grains with jam or honey

Snack: A banana

Lunch: Spelled salad with legumes, vegetables and a side of spinach

Snack: 6 nuts

Dinner: Warm octopus, zucchini and chicory

Sunday:

Breakfast: a jar of natural soy yogurt

Snack: Pomegranate juice 100%

Lunch: 80 grams of mackerel / tuna in brine

Snack: 30 grams of hazelnuts

Dinner: 150 grams of white fish with simple cooking

Recommended to drink a glass of wine or good water.

Importantly, in addition to following an anti-inflammatory diet it is good practice to perform regular physical activity and sleep at least 8 hours.

An anti-inflammatory diet, along with regular exercise and sufficient rest can therefore bring many benefits.

Conclusion

You are what you eat' implies that certain foods can be good or bad for you. They are bad if they are inflammatory foods and good if they are not. If you are a doctor who treats inflammatory conditions, like neck pain or low back pain, wouldn't you want your patients to eat foods that help to reduce inflammation as oppose to consuming inflammatory foods?

This GUIDE begins with the premise that eating certain foods can actually make things hurt worse-increases inflammation-while eating other foods can actually help lessen pain and promote faster healing.

These are known as anti-inflammatory foods and they are closely related to competing omega fatty acids. Swelling, redness, heat and pain occur when tissue become inflamed. It may be overt, like a sprained ankle, or hidden beneath the skin, like in your stomach.

An example of inflammatory foods are those high in refined or hydrogenated vegetable oils, like potato chips and many baked goods. Refined oils and trans fats are used by manufacturers to extend the shelf life of their products.

They are notorious preservatives. On the other hand, olive oil, avocado oil and grape seed oil are natural and are known to be anti-inflammatory. Salmon is very high on the list of ant-inflammatory foods.

The reason has to do with the competing omega fatty acids. "A healthy diet contains a balance of omega-3 and omega-6 fatty acids. Omega-3 fatty acids help reduce inflammation, and some omega-6 fatty acids tend to promote inflammation

Now, red meats, such as a good, juicy steak, are high in omega-6 fatty acids. So, does that make it bad? No. It's extremely good for you. A good steak is loaded with essential amino acids and other nutrients.

It's just that the key to improving health and reducing inflammation is to balance the amount of omega-6 (e.g., nuts, eggs, poultry, cream, cheese, butter) against the omega-3 (e.g., salmon, tuna, turkey). The saturated fats contained in omega-6 foods compete with the omega-3 foods for vital digestive enzymes, like seagulls fighting over french fries on the boardwalk.

Along with omega-3's, omega-6's play a crucial role in brain function as well as normal growth and development." Anti-inflammatory foods include colorful, high fiber vegetables like sweet peppers, celery, raw carrots, onions, garlic, broccoli, cauliflower, cucumber, apples, pears, berries, nuts, grapes, bananas, citrus fruits and so on (omega-3's).

So here's my advice: Limit fatty animal products like red meats and dairy products. Instead, eat more lean cuts of chicken, turkey and fish. Olive oils and avocado can and should replace unhealthy oils from corn, soybeans, safflower, sunflower and other vegetable oils.

Sweets should be limited, including all bakery products like cookies, cakes, pies and breads. We all know that our modern diet of processed and fast foods tends to generate inflammation and other evils, like obesity. To counteract bad eating, give close consideration to the competing omega fatty acids.

ALKALINE DIET

The benefits of eating alkaline foods, a guide for beginners to help you lose weight, keep in form

And

live a healthy life.

GILLIAN WILLET

The information provided herein is stated to be truthful and consistent, in that any liability, in terms of inattention or otherwise, by any usage or abuse of any policies, processes, or directions contained within is the solitary and utter responsibility of the recipient reader. Under no circumstances will any legal responsibility or blame be held against the publisher for any reparation, damages, or monetary loss due to the information herein, either directly or indirectly.

Respective authors own all copyrights not held by the publisher.

The information herein is offered for informational purposes solely, and is universal as so. The presentation of the information is without contract or any type of guarantee assurance.

The trademarks that are used are without any consent, and the publication of the trademark is without permission or backing by the trademark owner. All trademarks and brands within this book are for clarifying purposes only and are the owned by the owners themselves, not affiliated with this document

Table of Contents

Introduction

A lot of people have been struggling to find the best diet program fit for them. One of the most common misrepresentations these people have is their desire to lose weight. However, they fail to put vital emphasis on how to be healthy. If you want to know the best diet that is perfect for you, then you better make sure it's a healthy one, and is not destroying your body.

Chapter One

What is the alkaline diet?

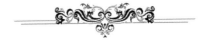

The Alkaline Diet, also known as the Alkaline Acid Diet, is a diet based on the consumption of food such as fruits, vegetables, roots, nuts, and legumes, but avoiding dairy, meat, grains and salts. Recently, this diet has gained popularity among diet and nutrition specialists and authors. There is still a debate on the efficiency of alkaline diet because there is no concrete evidence that it can reduce certain diseases.

As aforementioned, fruits, vegetables, roots, nuts, and legumes are part of the alkaline diet. This is because these food release alkaline after being digested, absorbed, and metabolised. On the other hand; dairy, meat, grains and salts produce acid after they are processed. Food is categorized as acid-producing or alkaline-producing based on its pH (power of Hydrogen) values, where pH 0 - 6 is acidic, pH 8 - 14 is alkaline and pH 7 is neutral (water). Hence, the alkaline diet refers to a diet having more alkaline-producing foods.

Alkaline Diet

Our blood has a pH between 7.35 and 7.45, which is slightly alkaline. The Alkaline diet is based on the pH level of our blood and any diet that is high in acid-producing food will destroy the balance. When the body tries to revitalize the equilibrium of pH in the blood, the acidity of the food will contribute to the loss of vital minerals such as potassium, magnesium, calcium, and sodium. The imbalance will make people susceptible to illness.

Unfortunately, Western diets are more acid-producing and on it people consume few fresh fruits and vegetables. Due to the advent of the alkaline diet, the standard of the Western diet has changed considerably.

Some diet and nutrition practitioners believe that an acid-producing diet may cause some chronic illness and the following symptoms, such as:

- Headache
- Lethargy
- Frequent flu and cold, and excess mucous production
- Anxiety, nervousness
- Polycystic ovaries, ovarian cysts, benign breast cysts

Although some believe the above conditions are the result of an acid-producing diet, and the consumption of fruits and vegetables is beneficial to health, some doctors think that an acid-producing diet does not cause chronic disease. Other than that, there are proofs showing that an alkaline diets helps to prevent the formation of calcium kidney stones, osteoporosis, and age-related muscle wasting.

Surely, you have encountered an alkaline meal program somewhere online or in some reading materials. What is an alkaline diet and is this diet healthy for you? This diet all started when experts tried considering the pH level of the body.

In a person's body, the environment can be acidic or alkaline. Once the pH level is high, then the environment is alkaline. In contrary, low pH means the environment is acidic. The body does not have one single pH level, rather it can differ depending on the location. For instance, the pH level in the stomach is different from the urinary bladder.

This diet is basically all about eating foods which can promote an alkaline environment in the body while not eating foods that promote acidity to the body. What could be the reason behind this program? To start off, foods that can promote an alkaline environment in the body are considered healthy. Examples of these foods include vegetables, fruits, soy products, nuts, legumes, and cereals. If you have noticed, these foods are also rich in protein, vitamins, and minerals.

Th other principle of an alkaline diet is to avoid acidic foods because these are foods that can make your body at risk for weight gain, heart problems, kidney and liver diseases. A few of the many acidic foods include caffeine, foods with high preservatives like canned goods, sodas, fish, meat, alcohol and foods with a high sugar content. When you come to think of it, an alkaline diet is not unusual for everyone, especially when talking about a healthy diet.

Real Deal with the Alkaline Diet

According to experts, acidic foods can decrease the pH of a person's urine. When the pH is abnormally low kidney stones tend to form. To counteract this situation a person needs to increase the pH through eating alkaline rich foods, it's that simple.

Since an alkaline diet means avoiding alcohol and any other foods with high acidity, it also means you will decrease the risk of developing diseases associated with an unhealthy diet like diabetes, hypertension, and obesity. Although no exact evidences can prove this, some researchers have stated that an alkaline diet can reduce the risk of cancer.

Things to Remember

In order for the alkaline diet to work, you must condition yourself to adhere to this diet program. When it requires you to avoid unhealthy foods and drinks, then you had better do it. Water is an excellent alternative drink for soda and alcohol.

In addition, so you will not have a difficult time figuring out which are alkaline and which are acidic foods, it is best that you make a list of each category. Perhaps you can research online on what foods are rich in alkaline and those having a high acid content. Alkaline foods are not that hard to point out because the majority of foods belong to the vegetables and fruits classifications.

When you choose to eat an alkaline diet, you are actually eating foods that are very similar to what mankind was designed to eat. If you look at what our ancestors ate, you will find a diet rich in fresh fruits, vegetables, legumes, nuts, and fish. Unfortunately, man's diet today is frequently full of foods that are high in unhealthy fats, salt, cholesterol, and acidifying foods

243

Although some people think that man's diet changed only recently, the shift from a largely alkaline diet to an acidic diet actually began thousands of years ago. Our original diet consisted of foraged fruits, nuts and vegetables, along with whatever meat could be caught.

As soon as man started to grow his own food, things started to change. Grains became a popular diet choice, especially after the development of stone tools. Once animals were domesticated, there were dairy products added to the diet, along with an additional amount of meat. Salt began to be added, along with sugar. The end result was a diet that was still much healthier than what many people eat today, but the shift from alkaline to acidic had begun.

It's no secret that our modern diet consists of many foods which are not healthy for us. Too much junk food and "fast food" has decreased the quality of our diet. Obesity has become the norm, and along with it a higher incidence of diseases such as diabetes, coronary disease, and cancer. If you want to improve your health and reduce the risk of many diseases, an alkaline diet can help get your body back to basics.

When foods are eaten and digested, they produce either an acidifying or alkalizing effect within the body. Some people get confused because the actual pH of the food itself doesn't have anything to do with the effect of the food once it is digested.

When more alkaline foods are consumed, the body can become slightly alkaline instead of acidic. Ideally, the blood pH level should be between 7.35 and 7.45. Foods such as citrus fruits, soy products, raw fruits and vegetables, wild rice, almonds, and natural sweeteners such as Stevia are all good alkaline food choices.

There are many benefits to shifting your eating patterns from acidic to alkaline. When the body is kept slightly alkaline, it is less susceptible to disease. It's easier to lose weight or maintain a healthy weight level on an alkaline diet. Most people experience an increase in their energy level, as well as a lessening of anxiety and irritability once they begin eating more alkaline foods.

Mucous production is decreased and nasal congestion is reduced, making it easier to breath. Allergies are frequently alleviated as a result of an alkaline diet. The body is also less susceptible to illnesses such as cancer and diabetes. Most people find that they just feel better, with an increased sense of health and well-being, once they make a conscious effort to adhere to an alkaline diet.

The Alkaline Diet Myth

The alkaline diet is also known as the acid-alkaline diet or the alkaline ash diet. It is based around the idea that the foods you eat leave behind an "ash" residue after they have been metabolized. This ash can be acid or alkaline.

Proponents of this diet claim that certain foods can affect the acidity and alkalinity of bodily fluids, including urine and blood. If you eat foods with an acidic ash, they make the body acidic. If you eat foods with an alkaline ash, they make the body alkaline.

Acidic ash is thought to make you vulnerable to diseases such as cancer, osteoporosis, and muscle wasting, whereas alkaline ash is considered to be protective. To make sure you stay alkaline, it is recommended that you keep track of your urine using handy pH test strips.

For those who do not fully understand human physiology and are not nutrition experts, diet claims like this sound rather convincing. However, is it really true? The following will debunk this myth and clear up some confusion regarding the alkaline diet.

But first, it is necessary to understand the meaning of the pH value.

Put simply, the pH value is a measure of how acidic or alkaline something is. The pH value ranges from 0 to 14.

- 0-7 is acidic
- 7 is neutral
- 7-14 is alkaline

For example, the stomach is loaded with highly acidic hydrochloric acid, a pH value between 2 and 3.5. The acidity helps kill germs and break down food.

On the other hand, the human blood is always slightly alkaline, with a pH of between 7.35 to 7.45. Normally, the body has several effective mechanisms (discussed later) to keep the blood's pH within this range. Falling out of it is very serious and can be fatal.

Effects Of Foods On Urine And Blood pH

Foods leave behind an acid or alkaline ash. Acid ash contains phosphate and sulfur. Alkaline ash contains calcium, magnesium, and potassium.

Certain food groups are considered acidic, neutral, or alkaline. They include:

- Acidic: Meats, fish, dairy, eggs, grains, and alcohol.
- Neutral: Fats, starches, and sugars.
- Alkaline: Fruits, vegetables, nuts, and legumes.

Urine pH

Foods you eat change the pH of your urine. If you have a green smoothie for breakfast, your urine, in a few hours, will be more alkaline than if you had bacon and eggs.

For someone on an alkaline diet, urine pH can be very easily monitored and may even provide instant gratification. Unfortunately, urine pH is neither a good indicator of the overall pH of the body, nor is it a good indicator of general health.

Blood pH

Foods you eat do not change your blood pH. When you eat something with an acid ash like protein, the acids produced are quickly neutralized by bicarbonate ions in the blood. This reaction produces carbon dioxide, which is exhaled through the lungs, and salts, which are excreted by the kidneys in your urine.

During the process of excretion, the kidneys produce new bicarbonate ions, which are returned to the blood to replace the bicarbonate that was initially used to neutralize the acid. This creates a sustainable cycle in which the body is able to maintain the pH of the blood within a tight range.

Therefore, as long as your kidneys are functioning normally, your blood pH will not be influenced by the foods you eat, whether they are acidic or alkaline. The claim that eating alkaline foods will make your body or blood pH more alkaline is not true.

Acidic Diet And Cancer

Those who advocate an alkaline diet claim that it can cure cancer because cancer can only grow in an acidic environment. By eating an alkaline diet, cancer cells cannot grow, so they die.

This hypothesis is very flawed. Cancer is perfectly capable of growing in an alkaline environment. In fact, cancer grows in normal body tissue which has a slightly alkaline pH of 7.4. Many experiments have confirmed this by successfully growing cancer cells in an alkaline environment.

However, cancer cells do grow faster with acidity. Once a tumor starts to develop, it creates its own acidic environment by breaking down glucose and reducing circulation. Therefore, it is not the acidic environment that causes cancer but the cancer that causes the acidic environment.

Even more interesting is a 2005 study by the National Cancer Institute which used vitamin C (ascorbic acid) to treat cancer. They found that by administering pharmacologic doses intravenously, ascorbic acid successfully killed cancer cells without harming normal cells. This is another example of cancer cells being vulnerable to acidity, as opposed to alkalinity.

In short, there is no scientific link between eating an acidic diet and cancer. Cancer cells can grow in both acidic and alkaline environments.

Acidic Diet And Osteoporosis

Osteoporosis is a progressive bone disease characterized by a decrease in bone mineral content, leading to lowered bone density and strength and higher risk of a broken bone.

Proponents of the alkaline diet believe that in order to maintain a constant blood pH, the body takes alkaline minerals like calcium from the bones to neutralize the acids from an acidic diet. As discussed above, this is absolutely not true. The kidneys and the respiratory system are responsible for regulating blood pH, not the bones.

In fact, many studies have shown that increasing animal protein intake is positive for bone metabolism as it increases calcium retention and activates IGF-1 (insulin-like growth factor-1) that stimulates bone regeneration. Thus, the hypothesis that an acidic diet causes bone loss is not supported by science.

Acidic Diet And Muscle Wasting

Advocates of the alkaline diet believe that in order to eliminate excess acid caused by an acidic diet, the kidneys will steal amino acids (building blocks of protein) from muscle tissues, leading to muscle loss. The proposed mechanism is similar to the one causing osteoporosis.

As discussed, blood pH is regulated by the kidneys and the lungs, not the muscles. Hence, acidic foods like meats, dairy, and eggs do not cause muscle loss. As a matter of fact, they are complete dietary proteins that will support muscle repair and help prevent muscle wasting.

What Did Our Ancestors Eat?

A number of studies have examined whether our pre-agricultural ancestors ate net acidic or net alkaline diets. Very interestingly, they found that about half of the hunter-gatherers ate net acid-forming diets, while the other half ate net alkaline-forming diets.

Acid-forming diets were more common as people moved further north of the equator. The less hospitable the environment, the more animal proteins they ate. In more tropical environments where fruits and vegetables were abundant, their diet became more alkaline.

From an evolutionary perspective, the theory that acidic or protein-rich diets cause diseases like cancer, osteoporosis, and muscle loss is not valid. Half of the hunter-gatherers were eating net acid-forming diets, yet, they had no evidence of such degenerative diseases.

It is worth noting that there is no one-size-fits-all diet that works for everyone, which is why Metabolic Typing is so helpful in determining your optimal diet. Due to our genetic variances, some people will benefit from an acidic diet, some an alkaline diet, and some some sort of diet that's in between. Thus the saying: one man's food can be another man's poison.

It is true that many people who have switched to an alkaline diet see significant health improvements. However, do bear in mind that other reasons may be at work:

Most of us do not eat enough vegetables and fruits. According to the Center for Disease and Prevention, only 9% of Americans eat enough vegetables and 13% enough fruits. If you switch to an alkaline diet, you are automatically eating more vegetables and fruits. After all, they are very rich in phytochemicals, antioxidants, and fiber which are essential to good health. When you eat more vegetables and fruits, you are probably eating less processed foods too.

Eating less dairy and eggs will benefit those who are lactose-intolerant or have a food sensitivity to eggs, which is rather common among the general population.

Eating less grains will benefit those who are gluten-sensitive or have leaky gut or an autoimmune disease.

Alkaline Water

One last point worth mentioning is that many people believe that drinking alkaline water (pH of 9.5 vs. pure water's pH of 7.0.) is healthier based on similar reasoning as the alkaline diet. Anyhow, it is not true. Water that is too alkaline can be detrimental to your health and lead to nutritional disequilibrium.

If you drink alkaline water all the time, it will neutralize your stomach acid and raise the alkalinity of your stomach. Over time, it will impair your ability to digest food and absorb nutrients and minerals. With less acidity in the stomach, it will also open the door for bacteria and parasites to get into your small intestine.

The bottom line is that alkaline water is not the answer to good health. Do not be fooled by marketing gimmicks. Instead, invest in a good water filtration system for your home. Clean, filtered water is still the best water for your body.

GUIDELINES

The alkaline diet is also known as the ph miracle, ph balance diet, or the acid alkaline diet, among other things. It based on the theory that everything that you eat can either cause your body to build up acid or to become more alkaline. For someone starting this diet, it can be overwhelming trying to figure out what is good (alkaline) and what is bad(acidic). This is why the alkaline diet guidelines will clear up some of the confusion.

There are many alkaline diet guidelines. The basic idea is certain substances are worse for the body then others. One of the alkaline diet guidelines is that you should attempt to eat 75-80% alkaline. Meaning that 75-80% of your diet is from the alkaline food chart.

Certain foods are considered more acid forming than others though. To give you an idea, here is a list of foods that are considered highly acid forming according to the alkaline diet guidelines: sweeteners (equal, sweet and low, nutra-sweet, and aspartame to name a few) beer, table salt, jam, ice cream, beef, lobster, fried food, processed cheese, and soft drinks. Here is a fun fact: cola has ph of 2.5. This is highly acidic. In order to neutralize one can of cola you would have to drink 32 glasses of water.

On the other side of the spectrum, there are certain food that are considered to be highly alkaline and when ingested help increase the alkalinity of the body. According to the alkaline diet guidelines, these food are as follows: sea salt, lotus rood, watermelon, tangerines, sweet potato, lime, pineapple, seaweed, pumpkin seeds, and lentils.

The alkaline diet guidelines say that drugs are extremely acid forming as well. Think about all those people who take some form of drug to ease their acid reflux. Little do they know their temporary solution is causing bigger problems for them in the long run.

There are many other alkaline diet foods and this was just an example. The more you eat them, the better you will feel. Many times people experience a period of detoxification when they switch to the alkaline diet. The alkaline diet guidelines suggest that you go through a period of a couple of weeks in detox to rid your body of toxins and allow it to adjust to this completely new way of eating.

LIFESTYLE

The low carbohydrate and high protein diets doing the rounds these days are an invitation to bad health. All athletes know that if a fit body is to be maintained one should steer completely clear of such diets. Not only do they result in extreme fatigue, they are also are a disaster where weight management is concerned. Choosing alkaline diets is the only way to live a healthy life, as well as shed those extra pounds.

Alkaline diets require one to follow a lifestyle completely opposite of the high protein low carb diets. The high protein diets leave the person following it fatigued and tired. It is for those who lead a stagnant life and want to shed some weight. But the weight that is lost comes back on as soon as one stops the diet.

With alkaline diets this is not the case. The diets can be incorporated into one's way of life and within days the results start to show. They require one to eat about 80% alkalizing foods so as to maintain the alkaline ph of the body at 7.4.

High protein diets tend to make the ph of the body acidic as opposed to its natural alkaline tilt. When the body's ph becomes acidic it attracts all kinds of illnesses and depletes one of energy. An acidic ph also results in rapid degeneration of the human body cells. That leads to a shortened life. One should stay away from these crash diets and look at achieving health and vigor by following alkaline diets instead.

Alkaline diets lead to the body's ph maintaining its alkaline nature. The various body functions are carried out smoothly and the immune system of the body stay strong. Under these circumstances one feels energetic as opposed to feeling fatigued. Also the weight shed like this stays off and most importantly the body does not fall sick.

In other words they help repel diseases as opposed to high protein diets which seem to attract them. These plans are also very good for those suffering from chronic diseases like arthritis, cancer, migraines, sinusitis and also osteoporosis. Following such a regime while taking medication helps fight these diseases off from the root.

Alkaline diets constitute mostly of fruits and vegetables. One should try to consume green vegetables and sweet fruits so that they make up about 70 to 80 percent of their total food intake. Lemons and melons should also be eaten. Almonds, honey, and olive oil are also high on the list of foods to be consumed for following alkaline diets.

Meats and fats should be avoided. All foods that are acidifying like coffee, alcohol, meats, and even certain vegetables like cooked spinach should not form more than 20% of one's diet. Alkaline water is also a must for everyone wanting to improve their diet. At least 6 to 8 glasses of alkaline water can do wonders for your body cleansing. Processed food is all acidic and also high in weight gaining substances and so should be avoided. Beverages like sodas are highly acidic and should not be consumed at all. It takes 32 glasses of water to balance out one glass of soda.

Chapter Two

Benefits Of Alkaline Diets

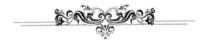

Wondering about the benefits of alkaline diets? Then you're not alone, because many people would love to learn more about this healthy way of eating, but they just aren't certain where to begin learning the real deal. That's why I'm giving you a guide to help you learn the truth about what alkaline diets are and the advantages that you can enjoy.

This nutrition program is called several different names, including the acid alkaline diet, the alkaline diet, and the alkaline ash diet. These names all refer to the same basic concepts, which stress fresh vegetables, fruits, whole grains, legumes, and healthy oils.

Why the Interest in Alkaline Diets?

Scientists realize that the breakdown of foods results in byproducts that can be either acid or alkaline, and that these byproducts can influence acid-alkaline balance in the body. The ideal pH of a healthy body is slightly alkaline, but the more acid-producing foods that are introduced, the more acidic the body becomes. An acidic internal system puts a person at risk for numerous health problems.

A great majority of the foods that the typical person eats today are highly processed, and they contain high levels of refined carbohydrates, unhealthy fats, sodium, and chemicals that contribute to health concerns. Sweet rolls, meats, and cream cheese all produce many acids when they are digested and absorbed. Processed foods are another type of product that increases the presence of acidic compounds. All of these acids are quickly released into the body's bloodstream, which creates problems as the body struggles to keep up its normally alkaline pH balance.

Experts say that you should have a pH level in the range of 7.35 to 7.45, but with the highly acidic American diet, it is difficult to maintain a healthy pH level, according to alkaline diet experts. These proponents believe that by supporting the body with the type of diet for which it was designed, better health and longer life can be attained. Humans are built for a diet of fresh produce and other whole foods that have been subjected to minimal processing.

What are the Benefits of Alkaline Diets?

According to nutrition experts, it is an acidic diet that is at least partially responsible for common problems such as premature aging and chronic illness. Health conditions such as arthritis and kidney stones are believed to be linked to diets that are known to generate excessive amounts of acids in the body.

Switching to a low-acid diet is believed to be capable of increasing energy, reducing mucus, relieving symptoms of irritability and anxiety, and may even lead to fewer headaches and infections. Scientists are now looking into claims that an alkaline diet has the power to prevent bone loss, muscle wasting, urinary tract problems, and kidney stones.

Ask people who follow these diets, and they'll tell you that they're healthier, happier, and more energetic than their counterparts who follow more low-carb diets. Plenty of people have found that their own health issues have either decreased dramatically or been completely eliminated once they adopted alkaline diets. Losing weight is also an important perk for those who incorporate whole foods into their lifestyles.

How to Get the Most Out of an Alkaline Diet

It can be helpful to refer to a list of specific foods, but generally you should attempt to eat an abundance of fresh fruits and vegetables every day. Salads are always a good choice. Make sure to drink lots of water, vegetable juice, or herbal teas. Avoid processed foods, fried foods, chocolates, foods that contain added sugars, and junk foods. Instead of adding sugar or salt to the foods you cook, try using healthy and flavorful herbs and spices.

The food that we eat today is totally different from what our ancestors ate and is completely different from what we are so accustomed to these days. How aptly said, "We are what we eat." With the advancement of technology, the types of foods we consume make us drag along. A view at the grocery store will shock you with aisles and aisles of processed food items and animal products. With the easy availability of fast foods nowadays, there is no difficulty in finding it in our neighborhoods.

Fad diets are being partly to blame for introducing whole new eating habits, and this includes high-protein diets. In recent years, consumption of animal products and refined food items have increased as more and more people leave out the daily supply of fruits and vegetables in their diets.

It comes as no surprise why, these days, many people are suffering from different types of ailments and allergies such as bone diseases, heart problems and many others. Some health experts link these diseases to the type of foods we eat. There are certain types of food that disrupt the balance in our body so that, during such instances, health problems arise. Unless we modify our eating habits, it's unlikely that prevention of diseases and restoration of health can be achieved.

Why Alkaline Is Important For Our Body

For a healthy body, the alkaline and acid ratio must be balanced, which is measured by the pH level in the body. pH values range from 0 to 14 and 7 is considered neutral. Any value less than 7 is considered acidic. Refined foods, such as meat and meat derivatives, candies and some sweetened drinks usually generate great amount of acid for the body.

Acidosis, a case of high level of acidic in the blood stream and body cells is the common index for the current different diseases inflicting many people. Some health professionals conclude that acidosis is responsible for the critical diseases suffered by many individuals nowadays.

An Alkaline or alkaline diet, which is normally present in our body neutralizes the high level of acid in the body to achieve an equilibrium state. This is the main function of the alkaline in the body. However, the presence of the alkaline in the body is quickly depleted due to the high level of acidic contents it has to neutralize and there is insufficient alkaline food consumed to replenish the loss of alkaline.

A Balanced Alkaline-Acid Level For A Healthy Body

As described previously, acidosis causes many health-related problems. A critical level of acid gets into our system, breaking up the cells and organs when not neutralized properly. To prevent this, one must see to it that a balanced pH is maintained.

To test whether our body contains a higher level of alkaline can be carried out with ease. This is done with the use of pH strips, which are obtainable from any pharmacy. There are two types of strips, one for the saliva and the other for urine.

Generally, a saliva pH level strip will determine the level of acid your body is producing; the normal values should be between 6.5 and 7.5 throughout the day. A urine pH level strip will show the level of acid; a normal reading should be between 6.0 and 6.5 in the morning and between 6.5 and 7.0 at night

High Level of Acidity Is Harmful for the Body

If you consistently suffer from fatigue, headaches and having regular common cold and flu, these symptoms indicate a high level of acid in the body. The effect of acidosis in the body not only inhibits the normal diseases that we know of, but other diseases that you may suffer from are caused by a high level of acid in the body.

Depression, high acidity, ulcers, dry skin, acne and being overweight are some of the things linked with an extreme level of acidity in our body. Not limited to these, there are other critical and serious diseases such as joint diseases, osteoporosis, bronchitis, frequent infections and heart diseases.

Even with medications, the symptoms may be disguised and continue to affect your health as the root of the problem has not been completely eradicated. Taking more medicine will only compound the problem as the anti-inflammatory medicine will add to the acidic level in the body.

Alkaline Diet - A Sure Bet To A Healthy Body

In order to reach the root of the diseases, our system's pH value must be maintained in a healthy state. Naturally occurring alkaline foods are able to supplement the lost alkaline levels in the body during the neutralizing process. By maintaining a healthy alkaline diet, sufficient amounts of alkaline are replenished in the system, thereby bringing the body back to the predominant alkaline state.

So, what are the ways to include an alkaline diet into our eating habits? The very basic first step is to reduce the amount of refined food intake. As we already know, these foods contain many chemicals which are the culprits in increasing the acidic level in our body. The next step is to cut down on the intake of meat and their derivatives and also the amount of liquor. The final step is to increase the amount of fresh fruits and vegetables, as they are naturally high in alkalinity.

Oranges and lemons are known for being able to convert acidic into alkaline after digestion and are absorbed by the body as part of a good alkaline diet. Generally, we must consume 75% of alkaline food daily. The higher the amount of alkaline foods we put into our system, the greater the neutralization of the acidic condition in our body.

Why It Is Recommended?

If you have heard of the Atkins diet, then the Acid Alkaline Diet is the complete opposite of that. The Atkins diet is a high protein, high fat but low carbohydrates diet. But such diets have a tendency to leave one low on energy and also they seem to be improper gastronomically speaking.

An acid alkaline diet on the other hand is not only useful for weight loss, but over and above that is extremely beneficial to the body's functions. An Acid alkaline, also known as an alkaline ash diet, alkaline acid diet and the alkaline diet, keeps the ph level of the body balanced and so safeguards against various illnesses. Even chronic diseases like arthritis can be not only prevented, but also cured if such a diet is followed.

The basis of a diet that is acid alkaline lies in the fact that our body's ph ideally should be at 7.3. This slightly alkaline level of the body's ph keeps all the vital organs functioning well, as well as the absorption of various minerals is optimized. When this ph tilts to the acidic side trouble starts brewing. An acidic ph level leads to almost all body parts suffering in one way or the other.

Now since our body needs to be alkaline in nature it should reflect in our food intake too. Foods that are alkalizing should be consumed much more as opposed to the acidifying foods. Translated into a simpler language this would mean more vegetable and fruit consumption and very low meats and oil intake.

If the body's alkaline minerals such as calcium, magnesium and potassium levels drop, so will its health, causing it to degenerate and its defenses to drop their guard. An alkaline diet protects that from happening. An acid alkaline or an alkaline ash diet comprises of 80% alkalizing foods and 20 % acidic foods. Since the acid alkaline ratio in the body should be one is to four, our food intake should be of a similar nature.

An alkaline diet is not only recommended to shed those extra pounds, but is also and more importantly a great means of regaining lost health and leading a longer and more disease free life. This diet is especially recommended to those who feel tired most of the time. Stress and a low energy level can both be done away with a diet that is acid alkaline.

Those who suffer from frequent viral fevers or those who have a nasal congestion most of the time can lead healthier lives if they have a diet that is acid alkaline. Weak nails, dryness, headaches, muscle pain, hives, joint pains, and many more such diseases find their answer in an alkaline ash diet.

A higher level of vegetable intake is recommended in an alkaline ash diet. Lemons should be squeezed into water drinks. Millet or quinoa is preferred over wheat, olive oil over vegetable oil and soups like miso are very useful for following an alkaline ash diet.

Lost health and vigor can be regained and many chronic illnesses prevented as well as cured if an acid alkaline diet is followed. It is a fairly easy diet plan, which should adapt you for a longer and healthier life span.

Benefits of Alkaline Diet for Diabetics

The human body is, to some degree, alkaline by design. By maintaining it alkaline we allow it to run at an ideal level. Nevertheless, millions of reactions of our metabolism yield acidic wastes as end products. When we consume an excessive amount of acid-producing foods and not enough alkaline-forming foods we aggravate the body's acid intoxication. If we let these acid-wastes build-up throughout the body, a disorder known as acidosis develops over time.

Acidosis will progressively debilitate our body vital functions, if we do not quickly take corrective actions. Acidosis, or body over-acidity, is in fact one of the leading causes of human aging. It makes our body highly vulnerable to the series of the deadly degenerative chronic diseases, such as diabetes, cancer, arthritis, as well as heart diseases.

For this reason, the biggest challenge we humans have to face to protect our lives is actually to find the right way to reduce the production, and to maximize the elimination of the body acidic wastes. To avoid acidosis and the age-related diseases, and to continue running at its highest level possible, our body needs a healthy lifestyle.

This lifestyle should include regular exercise, a balanced nutrition, a clean physical environment, and a way of living that brings the lowest stress possible. A healthy lifestyle allows our body to keep its acid waste content at the lowest level possible.

The alkaline diet, also known as the pH miracle diet, seems to fit the best for the design of the human body. This is mainly because it helps neutralize the acid wastes and allows flushing them out from the body. People should look at an alkaline diet as general dietary boundaries for humans to abide by. The persons who have particular health issues and special medical diets might better accommodate those diets to alkaline diet boundaries.

Alkaline Diet Benefits for Diabetics

The miracle alkaline diet will help improve the overall health of the persons suffering from diabetes. As it does for other human beings, an alkaline diet will help boost their body's physiology and metabolism, as well as their immune system. This diet will allow diabetics to have a better control on their blood sugar. It is also going to help not only in reducing their weight gain and the risks of cardiovascular diseases, but also in keeping their cholesterol level low.

In fact, the alkaline diet allows a better management of diabetes and, as a result, it helps diabetics more easily to avoid the degenerative diseases connected to their condition. So by following an alkaline diet, despite their health situation, diabetics can, at the same time, live healthier and extend their life expectancy considerably.

The alkaline diet rule sets general nutritional guidelines. According to this diet plan, our daily food intake should be composed of a minimum of 80 percent of alkaline-forming foods, and of no more than 20 percent of acidifying food products. Additionally, the diet highlights that the more alkaline a food item is, the better it is actually; and on the other hand the more acidifying a food product is, the worse it should be for the human body.

As for the glycemic index rule, it divides foods into four main categories with respect to their ability to raise the blood sugar. This ability is now measured by the glycemic index GI that ranges from 0 to 100. (1) Foods that contain almost no carbohydrates and that have, in consequence, a negligible glycemic index (GI~0); diabetics may take them freely. (2) Foods containing carbohydrates with a low glycemic index (GI 55 or less); people with diabetes should eat these products with some precautions. (3) Foods that have carbohydrates of high glycemic index (GI 56 or more); diabetics must, so far as possible, exclude them from their diet. (4) Processed foods; diabetics will need to consult the manufacturers' labels to figure out their particular glycemic index values.

Diabetics Top Best and Top Worst Foods

Intended for the people affected by diabetes, the 'Diabetics Acid-Alkaline Food Chart' divides foods into six categories. The list below goes from the top best to the top worst foods.

1. Alkalizing food items with GI~0. They are among the top best foods. Diabetics may eat them freely.

Asparagus; broccoli; parsley; celery; lettuce; carob; vegetable juices; mushrooms; squash; okra; zucchini; cauliflower; garlic/onions; green beans; beets; cabbage; raw spinach; lemons; avocados; limes; goat cheese; herb teas; stevia; lemon water; ginger tea; green tea; canola oil; olive oil; flax-seed oil.

2. Alkalizing food products that have a GI of 55 or less. People who have diabetes should take them with moderation, because of their glycemic index.

Barley grass; sweet potato; carrots; fresh corn; olives; peas/soybeans; tomatoes; bananas; cherries; pears; oranges; peaches; grapefruit; mangoes; kiwi; papayas; berries; apples; almonds; Brazil nuts; wild rice;

chestnuts; coconut; quinoa; hazelnuts; lentils; soy milk; soy cheese; goat milk; breast milk; raw honey; whey.

3. Acidifying foods with a GI~0. Diabetics should consume them with caution, being their acid-producing character.

Rhubarb; cooked spinach; pork; shellfish; liver; oysters; beef; venison; lamb; cold water fish; chicken; turkey; eggs; butter; buttermilk; cottage cheese; cheese; corn oil; lard; margarine; sunflower oil; wine; beer; coffee; cocoa; tea; mayonnaise; molasses; mustard; vinegar; artificial sweeteners.

4. Acidifying foods having a GI of 55 or less. Considering both their acid-forming feature and their glycemic index, people with diabetes will need to eat them with restraint.

Lima beans; navy beans; kidney beans; pinto beans; blueberries; cranberries; sour cherries; prunes; plums; brown rice; sprouted wheat bread; corn; oats/rye; whole wheat/rye bread; pasta/pastries; wheat; walnuts; peanuts; pistachios; cashews; pecans; sunflower seeds; sesame; yogurt; cream; raw milk; custard; homogenized milk; ice cream; chocolate.

5. Alkaline-forming foods with a GI of 56 or more. Because of their high glycemic index, these products are among the worst foods for diabetics. Therefore, people who suffer from diabetes need to avoid them.

Turnip; beetroot; tofu; potato with skins; figs; grapes/raisins; dates; melons; pineapple; watermelon; rice syrup; maple syrup; raw sugar; amaranth; millet.

6. Acid-producing foods with a GI of 56 or more. These items are too acidic and have too high-glycemic index carbohydrates. They represent the top worst foods for diabetics. Thus, diabetes sufferers need to cut them completely from their meals.

Chapter Three

Alkaline Diet And Cancer

As a result of the epidemic of cancer that has broken out in recent years, there have been great strides made in where cancer originated, how it grows in the body and how effective an alkaline diet and cancer regime has become. The definition of cancer allows the patient to have some control in the prevention and battle of cancer cells. By sticking to a primarily alkaline diet, this reduces, and actually quenches, the production of cancer and other diseases. Because of this, an alkaline diet has been found to prevent disease, while an acidic diet encourages disease and cancer to grow.

When you take the definition of cancer simply, it is 'a malformed cell.' This malformed cell can only reproduce malformed cells, and since the human body reproduces tens of thousands of cells daily, the answer is to stop that reproduction. The best defense then is a good offense, and that is what an alkaline diet does as it feeds the good cells, while choking out the disease.

The foods that are taken into the body typically come from two categories - foods that produce an acidic environment and foods that produce an alkaline environment. If you are taking a large quantity of medicines, this might cause your system to lean more towards the acidic, but it can be counteracted by consuming more alkaline-producing foods.

An alkaline diet is generally made up of alkaline-producing foods, so that the pH level is brought to a level of around 7.4. If you search online there are alkaline/acidic charts of all the foods. If you are just beginning this diet, make a copy of the chart and carry it with you when you shop or go out to eat.

In general, stay away from processed foods, fast foods fried in trans fat, any food made with white sugar or white flour, and all foods with chemicals and steroids.

These foods all feed cancer cells. If this is what your diet is made up of, check the alkaline food list and see what to be eating now.

Foods on that are alkaline-producing are vegetables, seeds, most fruits, brown rice and other grains, and fish. These foods can be mixed and matched to your own preference for at least 80% of your total diet, and then you add 20% of the acidic-producing foods, and the acidic foods are not all "bad." Foods on the acidic side are whole grain breads, lean meats, milk and milk products, butter and eggs, and this adds up to make an 100% alkaline diet.

To monitor your pH level once you have gotten started on an alkaline diet and cancer fighting way of eating, check any health food store for pH strips or litmus paper. There will be a color chart included to use and determine what your pH blood level is. For an alkaline system, it should register between 7.2 - 7.8. No two people are alike, so test your pH level about once a day as you get started. Then continue to check once a week. If you need to raise your pH level, eat more alkaline foods and use green supplements. An alkaline diet will prevent disease naturally.

Alkaline is most synonymous to its energy producing properties, hence alkaline batteries. It is this same energy generating properties that have been integrated into a diet principle. The alkalizing diet is also known as several other names, such as: ash diet, acid alkaline diet and the alkaline acid diet, is a method of consuming food that will leave ash residue, therefore prompting a process similar to catabolised foods. Catabolise or catabolism simply put is a manner of breaking down molecules into simple waste, therefore creating energy.

While the diet sounds complex in reality it is not. Alkalizing diets revolve around simple rules such as consuming several fresh fruits of the citrus family, legumes, vegetables, tubers, nuts and low sugar based fruits. Just about all the food consumed and digested once released to the blood is either converted into acids or alkaline. Exceptions to the alkalizing diet are fungi, sugar, caffeine and alcohol as well as avoidance of grains. The reason behind this exception is that these foods once digested will turn into acid.

The goal of this diet is to help maintain the body's natural pH level which is around 7.35-7.45. This practice ensures a stable alkalinity in the blood without stressing the body's acid base regulators.

Not to say that the body cannot maintain a pH level without this diet, while our system will automatically do this for us, it is however, maintained at a somewhat respectable level that can easily go from good to better or good to bad. What makes the alkaline diet essential is that it provides the body a different source of minerals like calcium from the bones instead of it having to dip into these said reserves.

As people age the pH balance fluctuates easily and can cause a decline in renal functions and the alkaline diet helps maintain the balance necessary in order to avoid this health decline in the future. Proponents of an alkalizing diet maintain that high acid producing foods can easily disrupts the natural balance, therefore incurring a loss in essential minerals such as magnesium, potassium, sodium and calcium when the body tries to restore its balance. some practitioners attribute this erratic activity towards the cause of illnesses.

Headaches, nasal congestion, sluggishness or lack of energy, anxiety, irritability, excess mucous production, nervousness, cysts, constant colds or flu are symptoms that alkalizing diet practitioners would attribute to a person with an imbalanced alkaline level. The diet is not widely practiced, yet as most physicians do not believe that the reduction of acid containing food such as meats, salts, refined grains and dairies and the increase of an alkaline diet is entirely beneficial to a person's health.

Furthermore, doctors will also point out that they are also uncertain that acids in an individual's diet are the main cause of chronic illnesses as claimed by alkaline diet followers. It is however proven that alkalizing diets do lessen the chances and help prevent osteoporosis, muscle waiting brought about by aging and the buildup of calcium stones in the kidneys.

Way too many people are facing terrible health problems such as cancer, diabetes, liver disease, high blood pressure, and more. Doctors over medicate patients and they become dependent on these medications. It is too bad more people have not heard about the Alkaline Acid Diet. This diet helps you keep an alkaline body and balance your body's pH. This diet is known to have cancer fighting properties and huge health benefits.

Ever wondered why the heart never gets a cancer? The heart might get affected eventually by cancer of any other part of the body, but we never hear of cancer of the heart. This is because the heart never gets cancer. The Alkaline diet is perhaps the only permanent way to prevent and rid oneself of cancer.

Let us understand what causes cancer and how an alkaline diet can prevent it. Each cell in our body takes in oxygen, nutrients and glucose while it throws out toxins. These cells are protected by the immune system. But as the body gets acidic the immune system gets overpowered by the toxins and the cell loses its capacity to take in oxygen and thus ferments. This cell gets cancer affected and is lost.

The next question is can cancer be prevented and cured by consuming a diet with less acid and more alkaline? Cancer cells lie dormant in a ph of 7.4 but as the body gets alkalized higher and the ph level reaches 8.4, these malignant cells die off. So the answer to cancer lies in an extremely alkaline diet. With the right consumption leading to a high alkaline body ph the cancer cells cannot live in that environment and die off.

Cancer cells being anaerobic cannot live in oxygen. They can only thrive in very low oxygen conditions. When the ph of the body is maintained by consuming an alkaline diet the immune system of the body stays strong. This leads to the cells getting enough oxygen and discarding their toxin waste. Cancer will neither thrive nor take birth under such circumstances.

How does an alkaline diet prevent cancer? Such a diet leads to a high alkaline body ph. This high alkaline body ph results in alkaline tissues in the body. Alkaline tissues hold 20 times more oxygen than acidic tissues.

Cancer cannot live in an oxygenated atmosphere. If the cells are oxygen rich they will prevent cancer. Therefore, while an acidic tissue will be an ideal ground for cancer to develop as well as spread, an alkaline tissue will destroy a cancer cell.

Having a lot of green vegetables and fruits along with alkaline water can save you from cancer. To give your body the best alkaline/acidic balance requires one to eat foods that are highly alkalizing while avoiding the acidifying foods.

An alkaline diet is very beneficial in fighting many diseases apart from cancer. Alkaline supplements are good ways to include alkaline food in your diet. Over cooking of vegetables leads to their nutrients being destroyed. Alkaline supplements make sure one gets enough alkalizing foods in a day. Also, alkaline water is a good alternative to ordinary water. So if you want your body to be cancer free as well as healthy and energetic adopt an alkaline diet and make it your way of life.

Chapter Four

Alkaline Diet And Weight Loss

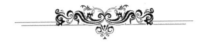

What if you knew about a weight loss program that would help you lose weight and feel younger? Would you try it? The alkaline diet and lifestyle has been around for over 60 years, yet many people aren't familiar with its natural, safe and proven weight loss properties!

The alkaline diet is not a gimmick or a fad. It's a healthy and easy way to enjoy new levels of health. In this post you'll learn about what this dietary plan is, what makes it different, and how it can produce life-changing results for you, your waistline and your health.

Are you enjoying a slim and sexy body today? If so, you're in the minority.

Sadly, over 65 percent of Americans are either overweight or obese. If you're overweight, you probably experience symptoms of ill-health like fatigue, swelling, sore joints, and a host of other signs of poor health.

Worse yet, you probably feel like giving up on ever enjoying the body you want and deserve. Perhaps you've been told that you're just getting older, but that simply isn't the truth. Don't buy into that lie. Other cultures have healthy, lean seniors who enjoy great health into their nineties!

The truth is, your body is a brilliantly designed machine and if you have any symptoms of ill-health this is a sure sign that your body's chemistry is too acidic. Your symptoms are just a cry for help. This is because the body doesn't just break down one day. Instead, your health erodes slowly over time, finally falling into 'disease'.

What's wrong with the way you're eating now?

The Standard American Diet (S.A.D.) focuses on refined carbohydrates, sugars, alcohol, meats and dairy. These foods are all highly acid-forming. Meanwhile, despite pleas from the nutritional experts, we simply don't eat enough of the alkalizing foods such as fresh fruits, veggies, nuts, and legumes.

In short, our S.A.D. lifestyle upsets the natural acid-alkaline balance our bodies need. This condition causes obesity, low-level aches and pains, colds and flu, and eventually disease sets in.

We've lost our way. This is where an alkaline diet can help restore our health.

I'm sure you're familiar with the term pH, which refers to the level of acidity or alkalinity contained in something. Alkalinity is measured on a scale. You can take a simple and inexpensive test at home to see where your alkalinity level falls, as well as to monitor it regularly.

Medical researchers and scientists have known for at least 70 years this lesser-known fact....your body requires a certain pH level, or delicate balance of your body's acid-alkaline levels - for optimal health and vitality.

You might think..."I don't need to know all this chemistry. Besides, what does the proper pH balance and alkalinity matter to me?" I know these were my questions when I first heard about alkaline eating.

We'll use two examples of how acid and alkalinity plays a role in your body.

1. We all know that our stomach has acid in it. Along with enzymes, this acid is essential for breaking food into basic elements that can be absorbed by the digestive tract. What if we didn't have any acid in our stomachs? We would die from malnutrition in no time because the body couldn't utilize a whole piece of meat or a whole piece of anything, for that matter! Make sense?

2: Different parts of our body require different levels of acidity or alkalinity. For example, your blood requires a slightly more alkaline level than your stomach acids. What if your blood was too acidic? It would virtually eat through your veins and arteries, causing a massive internal hemorrhage!

While these examples demonstrate that the various parts or systems in the body need different pH levels, we don't need to worry about that.

Our problem is simple and it's this.....we are simply too acidic overall, period. If you're interested in learning more about pH you can find tons of information on the web by simply searching the term.

The most important thing to know is this. When your body is too acidic over a long time, it leads to many diseases like obesity, arthritis, bone density loss, high blood pressure, heart disease and stroke. The list is endless, because the body simply gives up the battle for vitality and goes into survival mode as long as it can.

An alkaline diet is unique.

Many diets focus on the same foods that cause you to be overweight or sick in the first place. They simply ask you to eat less of those things, to eat more times per day, or to combine them differently.

In fairness to these diet's creators, they know that many of us don't want to make the bigger changes for our health. We like a diet that's focused on processed and refined foods, our meat, our sugar, alcohols and such. The diet creators are simply trying to help us make easier changes.

We've gotten used to eating this way, and it's not ALL our fault! Greedy food processing giants have a vested interest in keeping us eating this way. Profits are much higher in this sector of the food industry than in the production of your more basic foods like fruits and veggies.

So, again, YES...this diet is different. If those other diets worked you would you would be feeling lean, healthy and vital you wouldn't need to read this article. You wouldn't need a dietary change.

Here's a partial list of foods that you can eat freely in an alkaline diet:

- Fresh fruits and freshly made juices
- Fresh veggies and juices
- Cooked veggies

- Some legumes and soy
- Lean proteins and some eggs
- Certain grains
- Healthy fats and nuts

*You may be surprised to learn that some veggies and fruits are better for you than others!

You can consume limited quantities of these foods and beverages:

- Dairy
- Many common grains
- Refined foods and sugars
- Alcohol and caffeine

What's it like to be on the alkaline diet, and what results can you expect?

Like any change in diet or lifestyle, you'll go through an adjustment period. Yet because you're burning the cleanest fuel, which your body craves, so unlike many diet plans, you won't ever need to feel hungry. Plus, you can eat all you like until you're satisfied. You also won't need to count calories. And you'll enjoy plenty of variety, so you'll never get bored with eating.

Think of an alkaline diet as a type of 'juice fast' for the body. Only it's not so extreme. You're eating nutrient-dense, easily digestible foods that your body craves. When you provide all the cells of the body that it so desperately needs, your hunger goes away. And there's no need to worry about boring veggies, since there are tons of delicious recipes found on the web and in books.

With all the diet plans out there, why should you consider an alternative plan like the alkaline diet?

When followed properly, you can expect to melt the fat away more easily than with traditional plans. Many testimonials exist where people report losing over two pounds each week. (And that much weight wouldn't be wise in most diet programs.) Plus your skin will become more supple again, your energy will increase and you'll feel younger.

Plus, the alkaline diet does two important things that traditional diets don't.

1. It provides superior nourishment to your body's cells.

2. It naturally helps to detoxify and cleanse the cells, too.

These two facts are behind the reason why an alkaline diet works so quickly and safely.

There are a lot of crazy diets on the market that promise to help you lose weight. Unfortunately, if you look at the nutritional value of some of these diets, they are often severely lacking. If you need to lose weight, you should do it while eating a diet that is good for your body, so that you will become healthier instead of just thinner. An alkaline diet is a healthy approach to weight loss that will keep you energized, healthy, and motivated to drop the pounds.

Understanding the Alkaline Diet

An alkaline diet is different from other diets, because it focuses primarily on the effect that foods have on the acidity or the alkalinity of the body. When foods are digested and metabolized by the body, they produce what is commonly referred to as an "alkaline ash" or "acid ash." The original pH of the food doesn't factor into this final effect within the body.

In fact, some of the most acidic foods such as citrus fruits actually produce an alkaline effect when eaten. When more alkaline foods are eaten as opposed to acid foods, the pH of the body can be adjusted to an optimum level of approximately 7.3. While this is not extremely alkaline, it is enough to reap many healthful benefits.

Using an Alkaline Diet for Weight Loss

Many people attempt fad diets or those which promise quick results in an attempt to lose weight. These diets might produce results in the short term, but over time this can be a very unhealthy way to lose weight. Additionally, many people gain the weight back as soon as they go off their strict diet.

When an acid diet is used for weight loss and control, it is more of a lifestyle change. The results may not happen overnight, but it's more likely that the weight will not be gained back. An alkaline diet is rich in foods which are naturally low in calories, such as most vegetables and fruits.

Many of the foods that are high in fat and calories are also acidifying, so when these foods are removed from the diet, a natural and healthy weight loss will occur. These foods include red meat, fatty foods, high fat dairy products such as whole milk and cheese, sugar, soda, and alcohol.

Once you stop eating these foods, your body will be much healthier, less acidic, and you'll also lose weight in the process. Because the diet is healthy, you can stick with it long term. In fact, many people who start an alkaline diet solely for the purpose of losing weight find many other benefits. An increased energy level, resistance to illness, and an overall improvement in health and well-being are among the many benefits you can experience on an alkaline diet.

How to Start an Alkaline Diet

Many people find that it is easier to start on an alkaline diet by making small changes. Start by slowly reducing the amount of meat, sugar and fat in your diet, while adding fresh fruits, vegetables, healthy fats such as olive oil, almonds, soy products, and natural sweeteners such as Stevia. You'll find over time, your tastes will change and you'll actually start to prefer this kind of diet.

Recently, there have been numerous people claiming that you can use an alkaline diet for weight loss. Is this really true? Can a person really begin to experience weight loss simply from changing their diet to consume more alkaline foods? In this article we're going to show you if alkaline diets are effective, what changes they have on your body, and how exactly to utilize an alkaline diet for your best health.

How Your Body Handles Acid

So, why would anybody care about being on an alkaline diet to begin with? Well the reason is simple. As a population, we are throwing our bodies out of balance by ingesting toxins such as soda and animal proteins in mass quantities. As a result, acid is built up in such large quantities that the body goes into survival mode.

While acid would normally be processed and removed by the liver and kidneys, when too much of it exists, the body stores it in fat in order to preserve the health of your organs. The result is an unbalanced amount of acid and dehydration in the body. The body's homeostasis exists at a pH value of 7.3. Standard (neutral) water has a pH of 7.0. The ability to ionize water and consume an alkaline diet has great benefits for your health.

Alkaline Diet Benefits

But why is an alkaline diet great for weight loss? Well, a myriad of benefits have been attributed to maintaining your body's natural pH. Reversing the effects of chronic diseases such as diabetes, heartburn, angina, migraines, and arthritis are a few of the major benefits.

Freeing diabetics from their insulin crazed hunger fits has resulted in a large amount of weight loss. But, you'll see that even normal people have seen great weight loss as a result of an alkaline diet. When the body is freed of its toxic state, your metabolism is able to function more efficiently. Fat and proteins are burned and stored properly. Also, people have seen the benefits of increased energy and sex drive, allowing them to be more active and productive.

Optimizing Your Alkaline Diet For Weight Loss

If you are attempting to use an alkaline diet for weight loss, it is very important you know how to take the balanced approach. If you use alkaline water and alkaline foods in conjunction with a healthy lifestyle you will receive the "miracle" weight loss that everyone is raving about. Once you begin drinking the alkaline water on a regular basis, you can move from drinking water with pH 9.0 to pH 9.5 (for adults). Consuming a healthy amount of this high pH water is guaranteed to aid the body in returning to acid-alkaline harmony. Also, you should use the high pH water when preparing foods like soup and stews, to balance the acidifying animal proteins or other acidic aspects of the food.

In the above you have seen how you can use an alkaline diet for weight loss, but there is much more to be learned. In order to ensure that you are going to loss weight, it is important you learn about alkaline foods. Some of the most acid filled foods would be the ones you least expect. Many dairy products, for example, are very high in acid content.

Those struggling with excess weight see countless advertisements about thousands of weight loss products. Yet most of these people don't ever know WHY they are overweight in the first place. Many people like to have more energy throughout the day, but the snacks and caffeinated drinks that many consume are highly acid-forming.

What Excess Acidity Does Inside The Body

By creating acidity in blood, tissue and body cells, these typical snacks (as well as fast food, processed food, sweets, all yeast containing products, etc.!) may interfere with healthy energy production and often result in subsequent weight gain. The reason for that is the body's response to excess acidity: it stores acid wastes in fat cells to prevent them from attacking vital organs.

The over-acidification / acidosis of our body cells is the reason for many diseases, will interrupt cellular activities and functions, and is what causes someone to be overweight: to protect itself from potentially serious damage, the body creates new fat cells to store the extra acid. However, as soon as the acidic environment is eliminated, the fat inside the body is no longer needed, and literally melts away.

How To Lose Weight With Alkaline Food?

The body's internal environment is slightly alkaline, which is why it demands a diet that is also slightly alkaline. The body's entire metabolic process depends on an alkaline environment. Our internal system lives and dies at the cellular level, all the billions of cells that make up the human body are slightly alkaline, and must maintain alkalinity in order to function and remain healthy and alive.

Alkaline Food will make food cravings subside naturally, because the acidity inside the internal environment is neutralized through the alkaline forming elements. Once the inner terrain is alkalized with alkaline water and alkaline food according to an alkaline diet (=weight loss diet), the body is free to release the acid waste and burns off fat. In this way, your pH level will also be balanced, and every organ functions better, supporting healthy metabolism and making weight control much easier.

Some Good Alkaline Foods

Fresh vegetables, greens and grasses are excellent anti-yeast and anti-fungal foods, and green grasses such as barley or wheat grass are some of the lowest-calorie, lowest-sugar and most nutrient-rich foods on Earth (and contain high amounts of fiber).

Alkaline foods are mostly vegetables, especially raw ones. Most alkalizing are wheat and alfalfa grasses, fresh cucumber and some kind of sprouts. Furthermore, limes, tomatoes and avocado also have an alkalizing effect to our body, same as most kind of seeds, tofu, fresh soybeans, almonds, or olive oil.

What Are The Results Of The Alkaline Diet?

Once an alkaline diet is started, most people discover that their pH naturally becomes more alkaline. One gets to see how certain types of meals create a very acidic environment and learn to adjust their eating habits to better support weight control. When pH balance is achieved through alkaline food and alkaline eating habits, the body naturally drops to its healthy weight, food cravings will diminish, blood-sugar levels are balanced and energy levels will increase immensely.

Chapter Five

Alkaline Water

What Is Alkaline Water?

The concept of acidity or alkalinity of the body or of water is based on the pH scale. The pH scale goes from 0 to 14 and a pH of 7 is neutral. Anything with a pH below 7 is considered acidic and anything with a pH above 7 is alkaline.

The acronym "pH" is short for "potential of hydrogen." pH is a measure of the concentration of hydrogen ions. The lower the pH, the more free hydrogen ions it has. The higher the pH, the fewer free hydrogen ions it has. One pH unit reflects a tenfold change in ion concentration, so there are 10 times as many hydrogen ions available at a pH of 7 than at a pH of 8.

Our blood is slightly alkaline, with a pH of 7.4. Pure water has a neutral pH of 7, while natural water ranges from around 6.5 to 8.5 depending on surrounding soil and vegetation, seasonal variations, and weather.

Bottled waters marketed as being alkaline typically claim to have a pH between 8 and 10. Some are from springs or artesian wells that are naturally alkaline because of dissolved alkalizing compounds such as calcium, magnesium, potassium, silica, and bicarbonate. Others are transformed by a process called electrolysis that separates the water into alkaline and acid fractions. There are also expensive water ionizing machines marketed for home use.

Why Alkaline Water Cannot Turn The Body Alkaline

Marketers claim that their special water can turn the body alkaline. The truth is that they do not even understand the basic chemistry of how the human body works!

The main reason why drinking alkaline water cannot produce the health benefits claimed by the marketers is because one simply cannot alter the pH of the blood or the body this way.

Our diet, including the water we drink and the medications and supplements we take, can only alter the pH of our urine. Home test kits to measure the pH of urine do not relay any information about the body's pH at all.

The lungs and kidneys are the organs that regulate the body's pH, which is always kept in a very narrow range because all our enzymes are designed to work at pH 7.4. Even a small fluctuation, as little as 0.05 in our blood, can become life-threatening. That is why patients with kidney disease and lung dysfunction often rely on dialysis machines and mechanical ventilators respectively to avoid even a small disruption of pH balance in the blood.

In the stomach, where stomach acid is secreted, the pH is 1.5 to 3.5. It is a very acidic environment because the acid is necessary to break down the food and to kill all the germs and bacteria that may be in our food.

When we drink alkaline water and it comes in contact with the very acidic stomach, it is immediately neutralized because alkaline water has no buffers. A buffer is a chemical that can react with small amounts of either acid or alkaline substance to prevent changes in pH. An example of an alkaline buffer is baking soda (or sodium bicarbonate). Our lungs use bicarbonate as a pH-stabilizing buffer to maintain a constant blood pH.

Marketers claim that as the stomach acid neutralizes the alkaline water, bicarbonate ions are released into the blood, resulting in an alkalizing effect. This could only be true if the alkaline water effectively neutralized all the stomach acid, like baking soda would have done. But in reality, it is impossible for alkaline water to neutralize any significant quantity of stomach acid to create this "net alkalizing effect". As it happens, it is the other way around, the stomach acid completely neutralizes the alkaline water!

Alkaline Foods And Cancer

Proponents of an alkaline diet and marketers of alkaline water believe that overly acidic diets cause the body to become too acidic, which increases your risk of cancer. Although it is true that the immediate environment around cancer cells can be acidic, do know that it is due to differences in the way tumors create energy and use oxygen as compared to healthy tissues, not the acidic foods (such as meats, dairy, and eggs) that you eat.

Similarly, understand that their proposed answer to increase your intake of healthier alkaline foods like vegetables, fruits, and alkaline water can do nothing to change your body's pH. Veggies are good for you, but for a different reason - they are high in vitamins, minerals, and antioxidants which are anti-inflammatory and cancer-protective.

Alkaline Water For Detoxification And Hydration

Initial health improvements reported by people who drink this type of water can be attributed to the simple fact that they are drinking more water, resulting in improved hydration and detoxification. There is the placebo effect as well.

Moreover, alkaline water may contain higher mineral concentration, which is known to have beneficial health effects, especially when one's diet consists of mainly processed or junk foods that are very low in nutrients.

Alkaline PH-Level

The term pH stands for "potential" of "Hydrogen." It is the amount of hydrogen ions in a particular solution. The more ions, the more acidic the solution. The fewer ions the more alkaline (base) the solution. pH is measured on a scale of 0 to 14 with seven (7) being neutral. The lower the pH number the more acidic it is and the higher the number the more alkaline. For example, a pH-level of 3 is more acidic than a pH-level of 5 and a pH-level of 9 is more alkaline than a pH-level of 6. Drinking alkaline ionized water daily will help to balance and increase the ph-value.

As humans, a normal pH-level of all tissues and fluids of the body (except the stomach) is slightly alkaline. The most critical pH is in the blood. All other organs and fluids will fluctuate in their range in order to keep the blood at a strict pH between 7.35 and 7.45 (slightly alkaline). This process is called homeostasis. The body makes constant adjustments in tissue and fluid pH to maintain this very narrow pH range in the blood.

Diet is probably the most important change. Avoid the over consumption of meat, alcohol, soft drinks, caffeine, coffee, most nuts, eggs, vinegar, sauerkraut, ascorbic acid, cheese, white sugar and medical drugs. Add more ripe fruits, vegetables, bean sprouts, water, milk, onions, figs, carrots, beets, and miso to your diet.

Testing the pH Level

Testing saliva is the most effective way to gauge the body's pH. To test saliva: Wait 2 hours after eating. Spit into a spoon. Dip the strip. Read immediately. Use the color chart from the correct indication. An optimal reading is 7.5. This indicates a slightly alkaline body.

To test urine: Test a urine sample first thing in the morning. Fill a small cup with urine, and dip a strip into the cup. Read immediately. Results: 7.0 is neutral. A reading of 6.5 is slightly acidic. A reading below 6.5 is very acidic. Note: A reading of 8.0 or above, while common, indicates a body that is too alkaline. Urine is slightly more acidic than saliva. [from pH strip producer: Phion, Inc.]

About Balancing the pH

People with painful deposits anywhere in their feet may have a morning urine pH of 4.5! At 4.5 it may be safe to guess that a lot has precipitated again in the night. During the day, your body's pH may swing back and forth. The urine gets quite alkaline right after a meal; this is called the alkaline tide. Three meals a day would bring you three alkaline tides. During these periods, lasting about an hour, you have an opportunity to dissolve some of your foot deposits. But if you allow your pH to drop too low in the night you put the deposits back again. The net effect decides whether your deposits grow or shrink.

Items traditionally used to help nutritionally support the normal pH level of the body. The use of these items is a traditional use that is not intended to be prescribed for, to treat or claim to cure any disease, including diseases related to high or low pH levels. To alkalinize yourself at bedtime, choose one of these options:

Take calcium (pure calcium carbonate or coral calcium) equaling 750 mg plus 300 mg of magnesium oxide. The magnesium helps the calcium dissolve and stay in a solution. Taking more calcium at one time is not advised because it cannot be dissolved and absorbed anyway and might constipate you. For the elderly only one calcium tablet is advised. Take calcium tablets with vitamin C or lemon water to help dissolve (1/4 tsp. vitamin C powder; adding honey is fine).

One cup of sterilized milk or buttermilk, drunk hot or cold, plus 1 magnesium oxide tablet, 300 mg. (adding cinnamon is fine). If these two remedies work for you, your morning urinary pH will come up to 6.0, but if for some reason they don't, you may need to take more drastic measures. Take the supplements and milk earlier in the day and reserve bedtime for:

Get Balanced Bicarb Antacid (made from two parts baking soda and one part potassium bicarbonate). This potion may also be useful in occasional allergic reactions. Take 1 level tsp. in water at bedtime. If your pH reaches 6 in the morning continue each night at this dose. If it does not, take 1 1/2 tsp. Keep watching your pH, since it will gradually normalize and you will require less and less.

This is a short list of alkaline foods for pH balance:

Lemons/ Watermelon - pH 9.0

Bell pepper, kelps, mango, melons, parsley, papaya, seaweeds - pH 8.5

Apples, apricots, grapes, fruit juice, avocados, bananas, vegetable juice, peas - pH 8.0

Mushrooms, onions, almond, egg yolks, tofu, soy milk, vinegar, tomato, cucumber, coconut, brown rice - pH 7.5

These are a few common things that leave an acid ash in the bloodstream:

- Most tap water - pH 7.0
- Distilled water - pH 6.5
- Purified water, fruit juice with sugar, cigarette, tobacco, wine - pH 6.0
- White rice, beef, white flour, sugar, yogurt (sweetened) - pH 5.5

Acid pH:

- Reverse Osmosis Water, coffee, white bread - pH 4.0
- Cola, soft drinks, beer, hard spirits - pH 3.0
- Car battery acid - pH 1.0

Acid producing activities and emotions:

Overwork, anger, fear, jealousy, stress physical, stress emotional, Alkalize your body with alkaline diets and alkaline water.

- Stick to alkaline diets while minimizing intake of acid-forming foods
- Eat more greens and reds
- Drink at least 1.5l alkaline water every day

- Aerobic activities, yoga, tai chi, walking, swimming, rebounding and a positive mind are alkaline inducing.

Keep the body in an optimal healthy state:

1) The acid-alkaline balance, or pH balance or Yin-Yang balance in terms of Traditional Chinese Medicine, of the body is critical to optimal health. It is said that Taoists, Qigong masters and Yogis all live a balanced, harmonized and alkaline life. Acidified body, imbalance, and physical weakness caused by poor diet and soft drinks, stress and toxic environment are very common among most Americans.

Microstructure, electron-rich, reducing alkaline water is the smallest antioxidant in molecular size, thus drinking alkaline water is the simplest and most effective way to neutralize free radicals, acidic waste and carcinogen and flux out the accumulated toxins which are all electron-loving and provide best hydration to each cell in the body.

Positive effects of being alkaline and hydrated:

2) Blood is one of the fluid systems that are constantly trying to maintain a pH of 7.4 (slightly alkaline). Being slightly alkaline means the blood cells and body tissues are highly oxygenated, and in optimal state to neutralize and detoxify the metabolic waste and toxins and you will be in a state of:

- Vibrant healthy body
- Enhanced immunity
- High energy level
- Sharp mind and brain performance
- Shining looking healthy skin
- Positive emotional state

The pH balance is one of the most important measures to avoid disease at first and build up a strong functioning immune system. Cancer patients for example are always toxic (without exemption!) and most of the time eating the wrong food and having emotional stress or other stress related issues.

Terrain refers to the environment, the body fluids, humors. These make up 80% of the body and need to have a pH value of 7,2-7,6 so that the protits take on the form of life-supporting bacteria. Due to interruptions in Meridian Energy flow pH values can be different in various parts of the body. When the pH value changes the protits change into bacteria that can live in this low-pH, acicity environment.

Environment has 2 causes, Metabolism and Energy, both are interchangeable as 1st and 2nd causes. Protits are indestructible, they change their life forms = Pleomorphism. Energy is indestructible = change of flow in meridians.

For example, cholera bacteria requires pH 6 (assumed figure for demonstration purposes).

Cholera bacteria enters the body, which has 7.2 Protit will now change to a form that can live in 7.2, hence no outbreak of cholera. If body is at 6 cholera bacteria will florish, other bacteria in the body now also changes to cholera bacteria. That's the reason why some people get it and some don't. To explain the correlation between Metabolism and Meridian Energy which are responsible for the Terrain is a 100+ hour lecture.....

Nothing is a secret. 'Merck et al tests' every new antibiotic against its pleomorhic effect, so they know into what kind of bacteria the cholera will change (another harmful one as it lives in the same pH 6 environment). They know the only cure is to change the Terrain to pH 7.2, but this can only be done by metabolism, which requires good food and an undisturbed flow of energy.

>>

Pulsating Energy Resoance Therapy

(PERTH):

- Energy buildup and meridian (organ) balancing (PERTH)
- Complete body detoxification - naturally and soft
- pH normalization
- Treatment & Prevention of over 200 dis-ease conditions
- Increased cell metabolism
- Blood pressure normalization

Chapter Six

Eating Alkaline Foods

To become healthy you have to think healthy and this is why many people these days are turning to alkaline food diets. This is excellent for both your health and for your body. People on this diet have claimed they not only feel good, but also have more energy, an improved digestion and much less mood swings than before they started.

What Is an Alkaline Diet?

An alkaline diet is basically eating alkaline foods. The foundation for this diet is vegetarian. To get the best from this diet we will give you some guidance below.

- Vegetables would be arguably the most alkaline food around. Easy to buy and easy to prepare.

- Try to choose whole grain foods rather than processed ones because processed products do not have the same nutritional content.
- Some acidic foods such as limes, lemons and grapefruits turn to alkaline after digestion, so are very useful for flavouring.
- Other acidic foods also able to be used in this diet are coffee, cola, and broccoli, artichoke, asparagus, beetroot, spinach and cauliflower.
- Avocado, celery, garlic, ginger, onions, pumpkin are ideal vegetables to include.
- Tomatoes, pears, papayas, mango, apricots and apples can be included.
- Nuts to use are sunflower seeds, almonds, and walnuts.
- Oats, brown rice, and also almond and brown rice milks as well as coconut and coconut water can also be used.

Foods to Avoid

Red meat, poultry, dairy products and fizzy drinks are the foods that are the hardest to digest. Your kidneys have to take minerals which are vital for the body, like calcium and magnesium, from the bones in order to dissolve the acid in these foods.

This is not to say that small quantities of the above cannot be used to supplement and add variety to your meals. You will soon realise exactly what you can and cannot use, as your body will soon tell you.

Move towards this alkaline diet gradually. If you eat a lot of meat or love dairy foods like cheese, it may be best to try an alkaline diet meal 3 times a week to start with, so your body does not go into shock. Any diet has to be approached gently and once your body accepts the new foods being offered it will thank you by looking and feeling good.

As a guideline the pH of alkaline in our blood is measured from 7.35 to 7.45, and the level of acid is from 1.0 to 9.0.

Alkaline Diet Menu

By consciously controlling the acid to alkaline balance in your body, you are able to benefit from a wide range of health benefits. Increased energy and weight loss will be immediately noticeable to someone who is recently returning to balance from an overly acidic body.

By composing your diet of approximately 80% alkaline foods and only 20% acidic foods, you can return your body to its healthy, natural state. Also, preparing the acidic foods with alkaline water can greatly reduce their acidifying effect on the body. An alkaline diet works to reduce the stress placed on your liver, kidneys, and other organs by having an overly acidic (toxic) body.

Your Alkaline Diet Menu

Below are lists of different foods which are our top recommendations for having an alkaline diet. While foods which are acidic must be ingested for a healthy diet, they are too be lowered back to the levels which our bodies originally adapted to.

Alkaline Fruits:

- apples
- bananas
- blackberries
- dates

- oranges
- pineapple
- raisins

Alkaline Vegetables:

- broccoli
- cabbage
- carrots
- cauliflower
- celery
- eggplant
- mushrooms
- squash
- turnips

Acidic foods should make up no more than 25% of your diet. Listed below are the types of food which are acidic. Keep in mind that every category listed below has foods which are horribly acidic, but also some which are much more on the alkaline side.

Acidic Foods:

- meat

- cheese
- legumes
- grains
- nuts
- select fruits
- select vegetables

Top 10 Healthiest Alkaline Diet Foods

Ever heard of alkaline diet foods? If not, it is high time you do. Work pressure, home making, as well as maintaining personal and professional relations is taking a toll on everyone's food habits, resulting in more than 70% of the present generation suffering from acidity and heartburn. Every third person seems to be complaining of gastric problems, indigestion and acid reflux.

All of this is due to the imbalance in the acid-alkaline pH of foods that are consumed these days, where you simply grab something and rush to work. Fast foods, sodas and the like are being consumed left, right and center by the young generation, thus giving rise to deficiency in minerals, vitamins and nutrition.

Alkaline diets have been found to be extremely beneficial for optimum health. You can keep chronic ailments such as acidity, osteoporosis, and generalized weakness at arm's length with foods rich in alkaline content. Alkaline foods are important since the pH of human blood is slightly more alkaline. This makes it necessary that we have more of alkaline pH than acidic content in the body.

What are the benefits of Alkaline Diets?

Alkaline diet foods have a plethora of benefits such as:

- Improved resistance
- Vibrant temperament
- Increased Alertness
- Strong teeth and Bones
- Easy Digestion

Alkaline diet foods are vital to maintain the pH levels of blood at an optimum of 7. Alkaline foods are mostly vegetarian foods consisting of fresh foods and vegetables.

Listed here are the top 10 healthiest alkaline foods for nutritional benefits:

- Spinach and Greens - Spinach has been found to contain maximum benefits and is highly alkaline. It can be consumed raw or cooked with equal effect. Other leafy green vegetables such as lettuce, fenugreek leaves, basil, etc. also are extremely good as alkaline foods. They also contain a lot of minerals and vitamins as an added advantage.

- Cucumber - Raw cucumber is not only a zero-calorie vegetable, it is highly alkaline when consumed raw. It is delicious and contains a host of nutritional benefits. Cucumber improves overall digestion and keeps your skin fresh and glowing. It contains healthy alkaline water that helps in flushing out unwanted wastes from the body.

- Banana - Bananas can be considered a whole food due to its numerous dietary advantages. It gives instant energy and is hugely alkaline. In fact, if you are suffering from severe acidic problems, a banana diet can work wonders in reducing the burning sensation and indigestion remarkably. Bananas have healthy sugar content and can be consumed by anyone irrespective of his health condition.

- Celery - Celery is a delicious alkaline food that can help you immensely in keeping your pH levels at normal range of 7. When half-cooked, it gives maximum nutritional value and can be eaten as fresh salad too.

- Broccoli - Broccoli is one of the most nutritious and alkaline foods that has proved itself time and again. It is easily digestible and is a rich source of valuable minerals such as carotene and calcium. These minerals help in improving immunity and combat diseases in a remarkable manner.

- Avocado - This wonder fruit is a rich source of alkaline food and has an overall benefit in maintaining good health. Avocado improves your hemoglobin content and is extremely beneficial in restoring normalcy in a disease affected body.

- Capsicum - Capsicum, also known as bell pepper is a rich antioxidant and can be useful whether eaten cooked or raw. It is not only of high alkaline and nutritional value, it is also very delicious and adds taste to any dishes that are prepared with capsicum for flavor.

- Potato Skin - Although potato is found to be acidic in nature, potato skin is very rich in alkaline content. Raw potato juice is found to be very useful in reducing the acidic content in the stomach.
- Soy beans - Soy beans and soy milk are greatly alkaline and can be used as nutritional alkaline foods.
- Cold Milk - Cold milk is found to have high alkaline content and is often recommended to combat heartburn and acid reflux disorders.

Chapter Seven

Alkaline Diet Recipes

1. ALKALINE 'ACTIVATOR' GREEN SMOOTHIE

Ingredients:

- 1 lime

- 2 apples, chopped

- 1 inch slice of cucumber

- 1/2 celery stick

- Handful of spinach or kale

- 1 inch slice of pineapple,

- wheatgrass powder, 1 teaspoon

- water, as desired to thin consistency

-1/2 tsp spirulina powder, (optional)

-1/2 avocado, (optional)

Method:

Wash ingredients, place all in blender. Blend, pour, drink, enjoy! Activate your body's energy

Serves 1 (350 calories or 450 with avocado)

2. CREAMY DELICIOUS ALMOND MILK

Ingredients:

– 50g almonds or sliced almonds (it's best if you've soaked them for a few hours beforehand)

– 1 litre filtered water

– 1 tsp sunflower lecithin granules (optional)

– 2 medjool dates with stones removed (optional)

– a few drops of vanilla extract (optional)

Method:

Put all the ingredients in your high speed blender and blend for 1-2 minutes. Pour the milk through a straining cloth and into a container. Store the milk in the fridge – it will keep for up to three days.

You can use the almond pulp left over in the straining cloth to add into cake or brownie mixes.

Makes 1 litre (350 calories total)

3. CHIA CARDAMOM BREAKFAST PUDDING

Ingredients:

- 50g chia seeds

- 4 cardamom pods

- 10g hemp seeds

- 10g almond flakes

- 200ml almond milk

- 1 tbsp. agave syrup

- A few goji berries for decoration

Method:

Put all ingredients (except the gojis) in a bowl and mix thoroughly until all the chia seeds are covered well with the almond milk. Leave for an hour or two overnight so that the chia seeds expand and go gelatinous.

Remove cardamom pods and top with the goji berries. Serve and enjoy.

Serves 1-2 (400 calories total)

4. ALKALINE MINT-CHOOCLATE ICE CREAM SMOOTHIE

Ingredients:

- 4 very ripe, frozen bananas

- 4 small dates or 2 large medjool dates

- 1 tsp of carob powder

- 200ml almond milk

- A few sprigs of fresh mint leaves

Method:

Put all ingredients in a high speed blender and blend for 1-2 minutes. Add more almond milk for a thinner consistency or less milk for a thicker ice cream.

Garnish with a sprig of mint.

Serves 1-2 (600 calories total)

5. CREAMY KALE SALAD WITH AVOCADO AND TOMATO

Ingredients:

- 2 large handfuls kale

- 1 ripe medium avocado

- 2 ripe tomatoes

- Juice of 1 lime

- 1 clove crushed garlic or 1/2 tsp garlic powder

- 1 tbsp. agave syrup or honey

- 1/2 tsp. of paprika

- 1/2 tsp. ground black pepper

Method:

Wash and roughly chop the kale and tomatoes. Place in a large glass or mixing bowl.

Peel the avocado and add to the bowl. Juice the lime and add all remaining ingredients to the bowl. Massage all the ingredients together. Serve and enjoy.

Serves 1-2 (400 calories total)